AF842652

Galdós and Medicine

Hispanic Studies: Culture and Ideas

Volume **66**

Edited by
Claudio Canaparo

PETER LANG
Oxford · Bern · Berlin · Bruxelles · Frankfurt am Main · New York · Wien

Errata in *Galdós and Medicine*

p. 3 n6 l. 7	"description of Monina's death from diphtheria in *Leon Roch* in his *El Niño* (88)." [For "death" read "near-death"; for "88" read "188"]
p. 18 l. 20	For "Augustín Martín Niviero" read "Agustín Martín Niveiro"
p. 26 l. 19	For "insaciable" read "insatiable"
p. 26 n66 l. 3	For "insciables" read "insaciables"
p. 85 l. 8	For "fatal" read "nearly fatal"
p. 166 l. 23	For "death" read "near-death"
p. 214	*La familia de León Roch*, subentry *Monina*, diphtheria, death from: for "death" read "near-death"
p. 221	*Monina* (*La familia de León Roch*), subentry diphtheria, death from: for "death" read "near-death"

Michael W. Stannard

Galdós and Medicine

PETER LANG
Oxford · Bern · Berlin · Bruxelles · Frankfurt am Main · New York · Wien

Bibliographic information published by Die Deutsche Nationalbibliothek.
Die Deutsche Nationalbibliothek lists this publication in the Deutsche Nationalbibliografie; detailed bibliographic data is available on the Internet at http://dnb.d-nb.de.

A catalogue record for this book is available from the British Library.

Library of Congress Cataloging-in-Publication Data:

Stannard, Michael W., 1942-
Galdós and Medicine / Michael W. Stannard.
pages cm. -- (Hispanic Studies: Culture and Ideas ; 66)
Includes bibliographical references and index.
ISBN 978-3-0343-1825-9 (alk. paper)
1. Pérez Galdós, Benito, 1843-1920--Criticism and interpretation. 2. Literature and medicine--Spain--History--19th century. 3. Medicine in literature. I. Title.
PQ6555.Z5S73 2015
863'.5--dc23
2015002064

Cover illustration: Benito Pérez Galdós
Library of Congress, Washington D.C. (LC-USZ62-104648)

ISSN 1661-4720
ISBN 978-3-0343-1825-9 (print)
ISBN 978-3-0353-0695-8 (eBook)

© Peter Lang AG, International Academic Publishers, Bern 2015
Hochfeldstrasse 32, CH-3012 Bern, Switzerland
info@peterlang.com, www.peterlang.com, www.peterlang.net

All rights reserved.
All parts of this publication are protected by copyright.
Any utilisation outside the strict limits of the copyright law, without the permission of the publisher, is forbidden and liable to prosecution.
This applies in particular to reproductions, translations, microfilming, and storage and processing in electronic retrieval systems.

This publication has been peer reviewed.

Printed in Germany

To my wife, Becky.

Contents

Acknowledgements

I should like to acknowledge with thanks the help and interest of Rhian Davis with certain sections of this book, together with Susan Irwin and Jesús Terrón. My warm thanks are due to Professor Henry French of the History Department of the University of Exeter for his support in making the facilities of the University available to me. They have been invaluable, as has been the help of Aeronwen Cole, university librarian. An enormous debt is due to my wife, Becky, for her patient help in checking the typescripts and for her forbearance in listening to far more than she ever wanted to know about B.P.G.

CHAPTER 1

Doctors and Medicine in Galdós's Madrid

In 1889, Galdós wrote a prologue for a collection of stories about childhood by his close friend, the paediatrician Manuel Tolosa Latour (1857–1919). In it he compares their loves for medicine and for literature: "Certainly, you have more of the author about you than I do the physician; but your love of letters is no greater than the passion inspired in me by the noble science that you practise."[1] In this modest confession, he accounts for one of the features of his writing that distinguishes him from any other author of his time: a fascination for, and knowledge of, medicine that enabled him to describe in detail some of the most fearsome diseases of his day. Contemporary authors writing Naturalist-Realist fiction such as Leopoldo Alas (Clarin), Emilia Pardo Bazán and José Pereda included doctors and disease in their writings, but no one of his generation portrayed them with the detail and frequency that appear in the work of Galdós.[2]

Galdós was indefatigable in the depth and thoroughness with which he researched fields of knowledge for the backgrounds of his novels. Such

1 "Ciertamente, tienes tú más de literato que yo de médico; pero tu amor á las letras no excede á la pasión que a mí me inspira la noble ciencia que ejerces" (*Prólogo* ii).

2 Casalduero comments in the context of medical terms used by Galdós in *Marianela*, "Pablo has already mentioned the 'medical terms,' which he does not understand. In chapter 5, the novelist employs the vocabulary of mineralogy and geology. Now he does it with that of ophthalmology. [This is] a characteristic feature of his style, very unusual not to say unique in the nineteenth century. Baroja will follow him [in this] in the twentieth century," "Pablo ya habla de los 'términos de medicina,' que él no entendió. En el cap. 5, el novelista emplea el vocabulario de la mineralogía y geología. Ahora lo hace con el de la oftalmología. Escena característica de su estilo, muy raro sino única en el siglo XIX. Baroja le siguirá en en siglo XX" (Benito Pérez Galdós. *Marianela*. Ed. Joaquín Casalduero. 142 n. 7.)

detail is apparent in his descriptions of the financial speculation that occurs in *Lo prohibido*, the evolution of the Madrid textile trade at the beginning of *Fortunata y Jacinta*, and the world of fashionable ladies' attire that forms such an important element in *La de Bringas*. Among his contemporaries, Galdós impressed his friend and fellow novelist, Alas, who referred to him as, "curious about every type of knowledge, capable of penetrating the depths of many of them, if he determined that it was important to him."[3] Chonon Berkowitz later wrote that he used every type of resource to obtain the information he wanted, "he lost no opportunity to document thoroughly all the material he needed for his books, taking advantage of public libraries, private collections and archives, corresponding with people who could be useful to him, and consulting those who he used to call 'living archives' in the conference room of Congress."[4] Unlike the specialized fields of finance and fashion, what is particularly striking about Galdós's use of medical detail is the frequency with which it appears in his novels, both in major and minor characters. Medical oddities are apt to arise in the latter as a part of their natures, a feature of Galdós's technique of characterization.

This great flair for clinical description was recognized in the author's own time. In 1882, even before Galdós had written many of his most memorable depictions of disease, Benito Avilés, the editor of *La higiene*, wrote in an editorial celebrating the banquet held in the author's honour, "By virtue of his ability, on a par with being the leading Spanish novelist, Galdós is a great doctor. We have not seen, nor are aware of, so perfect a description of the horrors of croup [diphtheria] as he furnishes in *La familia de León Roch*; no one has described as he does the anguished scene of the death of a child."[5]

3 "un curioso de toda clase de conocimientos, capaz de penetrar en lo más hondo de muchos de ellos, si le importa y se lo propone" (22).

4 "no perdió ocasión de documentarse bien en todas las materias que necesitaba para sus libros, valiéndose de bibliotecas públicas, archivos y colecciones particulares, carteándose con personas que pudieran serle útiles, y consultando con los que él solía llamar 'archivos vivientes' en el salón de conferencias del Congreso" (*Biblioteca 10*).

5 "Galdós es á fuerza de talento y al par que el primer novelista español, un gran médico. No hemos visto, no conocemos una descripción tan acabada de los horrores del crup

In the following year, under the pen name of *El Doctor Fausto*, Tolosa Latour wrote an ample tribute to Galdós in *La Época*, emphasizing not only Galdós's wide scientific and medical knowledge but also his popularity among readers of the medical profession:

> He has affection for medicine and doctors. [...] *Augusto Miquis*, the distinguished physician of la *Desheredada*, is a portrait of body and soul; the scenes of *croup* in *Leon Rock* (sic) and the operation of *Teodoro Golfín*, the ophthalmic surgeon, are studied with exquisite care and described in a surprising manner; and finally there are not a few well-known doctors among his most assiduous and enthusiastic readers ...[6]

At Galdós's reception into the Real Academia Española in 1897, his long-term friend and ideological opponent Marcelino Menéndez Pelayo replied to his acceptance speech with a long account of Galdós's literary achievements. He paid particular attention to Galdós's ability to portray abnormal mental states, likening him to Charles Dickens, "who he resembles [...] in the richness of detail seen as if with a microscope [...] in the portrayal of unusual states of consciousness, the mad, sleep-walkers, mystics, visionaries, and fanatics of every type."[7]

---

como la que hace en *La familia de León Roch;* nadie ha descrito tampoco como él, el angustiosísimo cuadro de la muerte de un niño" (90, author's italics). As will be explained in the text, the relatively benign condition of croup (laryngo-tracheo-bronchitis), though described by Bretonneau in the early XIX century, was not widely distinguished from the much more lethal disease of the larynx, diphtheria, until later. Until then the term *crup* principally referred to diphtheria.

6 "Tiene afecto hacia la medicina y los médicos [...] *Augusto Miquis*, el distinguido médico de la *Desheredada*, es un retrato en cuerpo y alma; las escenas del *crup* en *Leon Rock* (sic) y la operación de *Teodoro Golfin*, el oculista, están estudiadas con exquisito cuidado y descritas de un modo sorprendente; y por fin entre sus lectores más asiduos y entre sus más entusiastas, cuenta á no pocos médicos de mucha fama ..." (*Siluetas* 3, author's italics). Tolosa had previously singled out for praise the accuracy of the description of Monina's death from diphtheria in *Leon Roch* in his *El Niño* (88).

7 "á quien se parece [...] en la riqueza de los detalles mirados como con microscopio [...] en la pintura de los estados excepcionales de conciencia, locos, sonámbulos, místicos, iluminados, y fanáticos de todo género" (125–26).

After Galdós's death in 1920, assessments of the medical portraits in his novels soon followed. Bravo Moreno in 1923 reviewed the portrayal of insanity in Galdós's characters according to pre-Freudian conceptions of mental disease, while Walton refered to Freudian ideas in 1927 when he discusses Ángel Guerra and Maximiliano Rubín (*Psicología* 177, 190), returning to a fuller Freudian assessment in 1948 (*Galdós* 11–12). Garma (1958), Elliott and Kerscheville (1940), and Ullman and Allison (1974) are also notable for their efforts to portray Galdós as a Freudian *avant la lettre*. Iglesias (2006) classifies Maximiliano Rubín's mental illness according to more recent diagnostic categories. Several characters in *Fortunata y Jacinta* are studied by Larsen (1996, 1998, 2006), while Gordon essays the medical background of *La desheredada*. A broader examination of the background of medicine as it appears in the Realist novel is to be found in the work of Pérez Bautista (1972), Granjel and López Piñero (1970–71), the latter also with García Ballester and Faus Sevilla (1964). Dissertations that have appeared on medicine and physicians in Galdós include those of Boix Martínez (1994), García Lisbona (1992), Smith (1977), Vozmediano Hidalgo (1981), and Willey (1964).

Unsurprisingly the majority of studies of medicine in Galdós have been made from a variety of literary perspectives, the few exceptions including Barbón-García *et al.*, and Álvaro and Martín del Burgo. There appear to be few studies that have looked in depth at the ideas current in medicine at the time that Galdós wrote.[8] Similarly absent is a study of specific texts from which he may have drawn, directly or indirectly, in his depictions of disease in his characters. This may relate to the apparent paucity among students of Galdós of those with medical training and an interest in nineteenth-century

8 Bell comments, "A great deal of Galdós criticism has, quite rightly, made much of intertextual references in Don Benito's work, but with regard to the presence of non-fictional, and specifically scientific works, there has been a noticeable absence of research or even interest. Perhaps this is due in part to the fact that literary critics tend to judge scientific works to be outside their remit, rather than viewing them as cultural artefacts, that are just as likely to have a bearing on the creativity of a writer as the work of other novelists." Bell registers, "medical science" as a partial exception, "insofar as it relates to the more radical naturalist novel" (180).

medicine. Taking this into account and bearing in mind my own training in medicine, this study has been undertaken in order to draw attention to this neglected aspect of Galdós's intellectual background. For it is clear that Galdós took medicine very seriously, and at least one writer on medicine in the novels goes as far as to assert that he would really have liked to have been a doctor, and that his passion for medicine, "was almost the consolation of a frustrated vocation: his [vocation] for medicine."[9]

Galdós's realistic descriptions of disease can invite medical analysis as if they were clinical pictures, and Ribbans expresses an ambivalent view as to how this temptation should be addressed. On the one hand he advises, "Care must be exercised in treating characters as medical case-histories and in particular in speculating beyond what is given in the text," while on the other he admits that, "At the same time medical evidence can be very useful in elucidating, verifying or assessing the information provided."[10] The essence of Ribbans' counsel revolves about the information provided in Galdós's text, attentive study of which frequently throws additional light upon the conditions he describes. This is especially true if his text is approached with some knowledge of the medical background of his time. Much can be elucidated from the information he provides, as the following chapters illustrate.

The changes in medicine that took place in Galdós's lifetime were enormous. At his birth in 1843, the role of micro-organisms in human disease had barely been recognized and laboratory medicine was in its infancy. By the time of his death in 1920, medicine had entered a recognizably modern era following the discovery of X-rays and viruses, and the development of blood transfusion and the electrocardiogram. The organisms responsible for the great epidemic and endemic diseases: tuberculosis, typhoid, whooping cough, tetanus, diphtheria, cholera, leprosy and syphilis were all discovered in the course of his lifetime. Galdós was aged twenty-four when Lister developed the technique of surgical antisepsis with carbolic

9 "una afición sincera, un casi consuelo a una frustrada vocación: la suya por la medicina" (Rubin 78).

10 *Pérez* 93.

acid that later evolved into the modern practice of asepsis. Lister's work greatly increased the scope and safety of surgery, especially in conjunction with inhalational anaesthesia adopted from the 1840s onwards. Galdós was a personal friend of several Madrid surgeons who were prominent in introducing these innovations in Spain.[11] He was well-placed to learn about these medical advances.

Some medical discoveries may take years, if not decades, to be accepted in medical practice. This was especially true in Spain where almost all the major advances in medicine of Galdós's time were first developed outside the country.[12] The *Guerra de Independencia*,[13] three Carlist civil wars and the Revolution of 1868 left the country ill-equipped to invest in scientific research.[14] Added to this, the tradition of xenophobic ultra-conservatism

11 According to Salvador de Madariaga, Enrique Diego-Madrazo spread the knowledge of antisepsis in surgical practice, which he had learned from Lister's disciple von Bergmann, while later teaching it in Barcelona (114). Alejandro San Martín pioneered the development and application of inhalational anaesthesia, vascular surgery and antisepsis, being acquainted with Lister personally (Herrera Rodríguez 390–401).

12 The striking exception to this rule is the Nobel laureate, Santiago Ramón y Cajal (1852–1934) who, building upon a school of histology in Spain, later became the founder of modern neurohistology. He was famously critical of the development of the sciences in Spain, "The chariot of Spanish thought lacks the wheel of science," "Al carro del pensimiento español le falta la rueda de la ciencia" (Marañón, *Ciencia* 485). In the context of medical advances generally, Rosenberg observes, "Changes in world-view are presumably always syncretic and gradual, not abrupt, self-conscious and categorical" (*Nightingale* 106).

13 *Guerra de Independencia* is the preferred name in Spain for what English-speaking historians commonly refer to as the Peninsular War (1808–1814).

14 Comenge comments in the context of factors contributing to the backwardness of Spanish medicine, "the rivers of blood and treasury of life that Spain has consumed in its foreign wars, in its unending domestic and colonial struggles [...] not for its prosperity, but for [its] mere existence as a poor, badly governed and little educated country," "los ríos de sangre y los tesoros de vida que España ha consumido en sus guerras con el extranjero, en sus inacabables luchas civiles y coloniales [...] no ya para su prosperidad, sino para la mera existencia de un país pobre, desgovernado y poco instruído" (x).

allied with the Catholic Church militated against Spanish scientists' attempts to adopt or develop new ideas.[15] Holding views linked with the theory of evolution after the publication of Darwin's *On the Origin of Species* in 1859, could be considered as grounds for dismissal as late as the 1890s. In Galdos's time, Madrid suffered more from diseases resulting from poor sanitation than any other Western European city. While new sanitary measures had been introduced from England in 1834 by Mateo Seoane, on his return after the death of Ferdinand VII, they had not kept pace with with the growth of cities.[16] Major movement from rural communities to cities in search of work resulted in population growth that far out-stripped facilities for the provision of clean water, and adequate disposal of waste. In comparison with cities abroad, and with Barcelona and Bilbao in Spain, Madrid also lagged far behind in industrial development with the result that most newcomers were unable to find regular employment.[17] This, in

15 Kaplan observes, "Spanish scientific and educational institutions were deliberately destroyed by the reactionary King Ferdinand VII when he regained the throne in 1823. Ferdinand re-established the Inquisition and drove into exile the liberals and progressives, among whom were physicians and leading scientists. The ruthlessness of the conservative political forces accounted for the dark age of Spanish science at mid-century. Phrenologists and physicians interested in forensic medicine were especially persecuted because of their emphasis on the physical rather than philosophical processes of the mind and their lack of interest in questions of morality" (525–26).

16 The introduction of sanitary ideas from England into Spain by Mateo Seoane is the subject of a study by López Piñero. Continuing deficiencies in sanitation in 1888–92 are reviewed by Fernández, *Epidemias* 211.

17 From the perspective of industrialized Cataluña in 1887, the lawyer and journalist Valentí Almirall judges the only industry of Madrid to be one of governmental administration, from whence all great personal fortunes were derived. "Its industry is almost non-existent and its commerce limited to providing for the necessities of local consumption (69) […] At first sight, Madrid seems to be a population of the unemployed (70) […] in Madrid there is no true working class, but there is no true middle-class either. The bourgeois who live by their labour, their commerce or their industry are squeezed out of all forms of social life by officialdom, which overwhelms them in number and influence. […] the political parasites have invented a different profitable source of income: graft" (72), "Su industria es casi nula y su comercio se

turn, led to gross overcrowding in fearfully unhealthy suburbs, *barrios*, from which disease, prostitution and crime threatened to extend to the rest of the capital.

The consequences for the health of most *madrileños* were dire. Mortality statistics compiled from the middle of the century onwards showed the highest infant mortality rates in any Western European city, with the highest mortality for those of adult years.[18] Any newcomer to Madrid, like Galdós coming from the relatively salubrious port city of Las Palmas, cannot but have been very aware of the plight of his fellow citizens. As a journalist with zeal to explore Madrid society, Galdós must have witnessed much of its poverty and disease; he observed firsthand the major outbreaks of cholera that spread to the capital in 1865 and 1884–85.

Struggling with Madrid's inadequate health statistics, Francisco Méndez Álvaro, president of the *Sociedad Española de Higiene* founded in 1882, drew upon figures compiled in Berlin, London and Paris as he and other members of the new society attempted to account for the mortality rates seen in Madrid in that year. The rate in 1882 was twice that of English and French capitals (*Actividad* 9) with a marked increase since previous years in deaths from smallpox, measles, diphtheria, and tuberculosis and, above all, from acute respiratory infections (5). Members of the Society suggested that the high altitude and harsh winter winds of the capital contributed to this mortality, in association with the permeable, porous soil that was thought to favour the development of epidemics. They highlight the inadequacy of the city's system of drains for removing factory and

---

limita á cubrir las necesidades del consumo local (69)... Al primer golpe de vista Madrid parece una población de desocupados (70) ... [...] en Madrid no hay una verdadera clase obrera; pero tampoco hay una verdadera burguesía. Los burgueses que viven de su trabajo, de su comercio o de su industria se ven ahogados en todas las manifestaciones de la vida social por la burguesía oficial, que los aplasta por número y por influencia [...] los vividores políticos han inventado otra substanciosa fuente de ingresos: el chanchullo" (72).

18 Fernández, *Epidemias* 212.

private waste, which had not kept pace with the city's population.[19] The group refers to what they regard as the model Public Health Act in England of 1875 and asks rhetorically how long it will be before similarly mandated measures for community health infrastructure are seen in Madrid (20). The editor of *La higiene*, Benito Avilés, associates a "fever" of overbuilding with the accompanying need to move large quantities of earth contaminated by open latrines, which he relates to the "terrifying mortality," *espantosa mortalidad*, of the years between 1880 and 1891, particularly due to typhoid fever. He also notes the deficient system of sewers of Madrid, and the inefficiency and irregularity of their inspection (*Higiene* 826). Hygienists were even more discouraged by the lack of significant progress in the decades between 1880 and 1900. Physicians of the city's *Beneficencia Municipal*, such as Fatás y Montes, in his 1903 analysis of the causes of infant mortality, high in comparison with other cities, makes the same complaints about governmental indifference to public health that had been aired twenty years earlier:

> Associated with the increased mortality as a result of infectious diseases [are] the bad organization of Madrid's sanitary system, the failure to fulfil the regulations designed to prevent [those diseases], the apathy of authorities in undertaking reforms of any kind that fall within the sphere of public health and the failure [of individuals] to observe the norms of personal hygiene.[20]

Echoing the deficiencies of the sanitary corps of the medical profession, Ángel Pulido, by 1902 Director General for Public Health, sternly rebuked

19 "The entire system for the drainage of foul water, be it from industrial or domestic usage or for rain run-off, is extremely deficient, and constitutes one of the gravest dangers to the health of the populace," "El sistema entero de evacuación de las aguas inmundas, de las que han servido para la industria ó usos domésticos y de las de lluvia, es defectuosísimo, y constituye uno de los más graves peligros para la salud del vecindario" (27).

20 "Concurren á la crecida mortalidad por enfermedades infecciosas la mala organización sanitaria de Madrid, el incumplimiento de las disposiciones que tienden á prevenir aquellas, la apatía de las autoridades para emprender las reformas de toda clase que son del dominio de la hygiene pública y la inobservancia de los preceptos de higiene individual" (134).

the nation's colleges of medicine and pharmacy for the shortcomings of public health physicians deploring "the backward state in which our national, provincial and municipal sanitary doctors find themselves, and the little understanding that the classes of the nation's society have of so important a branch of public life."[21]

A root cause appears to have been the reluctance of successive governments to delegate administration of public health and sanitation to the medical profession, starving them of both money and the necessary impetus for reform. Comenge writes in 1914:

> The power awarded to political bosses and mayors, their subordination of sanitary committees and inspectors, who only had responsabilities and difficulties, and, to crown it all, the weight of political alliances in decisions of [public] hygiene, provide eloquent explanations for the fruitlessness of the work of sanitary legislation. And this sterility was not restricted to the generations of the mid-century, it continued and continues at present in the absence of coherence and authority in public health administration and the gulf between the community and public health. We descend into a sad and shameful situation, not only in the face of exotic infectous diseases, but in the struggle against preventable illnesses (smallpox) and inhuman violations, the adulteration of foodstuffs and insanitary housing, for example.[22]

Faced with such daunting medical problems, a new generation of physicians arose in the wake of liberalizing reforms in medical education that followed the Revolution of 1868. Largely liberal in politics, anxious to escape the

21 "el estado de atraso en que se hallan nuestros servicios sanitarios oficiales (nacionales, provincials y municipals), y la poca ilustración que manifiestan en ramo tan principal de la vida pública las clases sociales de la Nación" (*Dirección* 879).

22 "La preponderancia otorgada a los jefes politicos y alcaldes, la supeditación a éstos de juntas e inspectores sanitarios, quienes sólo tuvieron responsabilidades y molestias, y, por fin, la pesadumbre de la amistad política en las decisiones higiénicas, dan argumentos explicitivos de lo infructuoso de la tarea legislativo-sanitaria. Y tal esterilidad no fue exclusiva de las generaciones de mediados de la centuria, persistían ella y subsiste en días presentes en que la falta de trabazón y de autoridad en el organismo higiénico y el divorcio entre el pueblo y la sanidad, nos sumen en situación afrentosa y triste, no ya sólo ante contagios exóticos, sino en la lucha contra dolencias evitables (viruela) y trasgresiones inhumanas, adulteración de substancias y viviendas insanas, por ejemplo" (401).

restrictions of religious conservatism and to embrace medical advances emanating from France, Germany and England, this generation included a remarkable group that fell under the influence of the charismatic José María Esquerdo (1842–1912). This Valencian of humble origins lectured in general pathology and mental diseases in the free medical school created after the Revolution. In the face of many privations, he had become a disciple of the leading medico-legal scholar in Spain, Pedro Mata.[23] Born in the year before Galdós, his life would intersect directly and indirectly with the author's until his death in 1912. He shared the successful Socialist-Republican political platform with Galdós in 1910. Esquerdo was the best-known Madrid *alienista* of his day;[24] Galdós mentions him by name twice in his novels.[25]

23 Born in Villajoyosa (Alicante), Esquerdo was orphaned and brought up by an uncle, a one-time Augustinian friar. As a child, he was deeply impressed by the sight of a lunatic being beaten in an asylum. After training in medicine in Valencia and Madrid, he joined the staff of the *Hospital Provincial*. He led a vigorous campaign to have criminal insanity recognized by the courts under the slogan of *Locos que no lo parecen*. He founded a private asylum at Carabanchel in 1877 and another in Villajoyosa. He became leader of the Republican Party on the death of Ruíz Zorilla in 1895 and was active in politics for the rest of his life (Eleizegui).

24 Alienism (*alienismo, aliénisme*) arose in France as a result of pioneers such as Pinel and Esquirol. Reflecting the positivist view of its time, it was predicated on the belief that a structural, neurological abnormality underlay mental disease. This contrasts with the later psychodynamic theories of Freud and his contemporaries in Vienna that came to dominate psychiatric thought after 1890. When the search for structural abnormality at autopsy failed to reveal anything in many cases, an alternative biological narrative of degeneration dominated French *aliénisme* for the rest of the XIX century. For discussions of the theory of degeneration, see Pick, and Stannard (*Degeneration*).

25 *Lo prohibido* (I.vi.153) and *Fortunata y Jacinta II* (I.xi.323).

While Esquerdo's written contributions to psychiatry were minimal,[26] his charismatic and generous personality[27] inspired the loyalty of a talented band of disciples each of whom would produce original work.[28] The most important of these, from the point of view of Galdós, was Tolosa Latour with whom, from the early 1880s onwards, he maintained a close friendship based on shared interests in literature, theatre and medicine. Son of a Spanish father and French mother, Tolosa put his bilingual skills to work in the translation of French medical texts. Correspondence that survives between the two documents the closeness of their friendship.[29] Galdós later wrote of the innumerable evenings that they had spent in each other's company, especially after Tolosa's marriage to the actress Eliza Mendoza (*Memorias* 94). Their correspondence documents the interchange of medical information on topics that captured Galdós's interest, and there can be little doubt that he learned much about the medicine of his day from the conversations of those many, sadly unrecorded, evenings.[30]

26 Huertas comments, "Although Esquerdo and Vera are widely recognized and quoted authors as genuine representatives of the so-called Madrid 'school,' there scarcely exist investigations of the time that increased the depth of understanding in Spanish psychiatry of the XIX century, either in their work or its real significance," "Aunque Esquerdo y Vera son autores profusamente citados y reconocidos como genuinos representantes de la llamada 'escuela' madrileña, apenas existen investigaciones históricas que hayan profundizado ni en su obra, ni en el significado real de la misma en el contexto de la psiquiatría española del XIX" (*Organizar* 77). For his tendency to have others report or transcribe his rhetoric-laden conferences, Villasante more bluntly calls him, "fundamentally illiterate," "fundamentalmente ágrafo" (*Introducción* 65).

27 Marañón refers to his "beautiful and ingenuous spirit of generosity [both] lay and liberal," "aquel hermoso y cándido espíritu de generosidad liberal y laica" (*Psiquiatras* 83).

28 "he organized a fervent group of followers [...] from which developed men who were later outstanding in Medicine in their own right," "organizó un apostolado [...] y de él formaron parte figuras que luego brillaron con intensa luz propia en el campo de la Medicina" (Manuel Ortega 64–65).

29 "A long-lived friendship of great intimacy," "una amistad de gran intimidad y duración" (Schmidt 11).

30 There appears to be no biography of Tolosa Latour, whose similarly named nephew and great nephew followed him in the practice of paediatrics. He is remembered in

A friend of Tolosa with a successful career as a prolific medical journalist, author and politician was Ángel Pulido (1852–1932), according to his son the most favoured by Esquerdo among his students.[31] Pulido was a tireless writer and campaigner in support of improving public health, of raising standards within the medical profession, and supporting Esquerdo's crusade to have criminal insanity recognized by the Spanish judiciary. Together with Tolosa, Pulido published a highly laudatory account of Esquerdo's asylums at Carabanchel Alto and Villajoyosa, *De Carabanchel al paraíso (recuerdos de un manicomio)*, in *El siglo médico* in 1882.[32] His travels to medical institutions and conferences abroad made him conversant with medical advances in and outside Spain. He visited Valencia in

---

obituaries especially for legislation (*la Ley de Protección a la Infancia, "la ley Tolosa"* 1904) that mandated legal protection for abandoned children and their freedom from child labour. A memorial bust of him is located close to the rose garden of the Retiro Park in Madrid, not far from the statue of Galdós.

31 Ángel Pulido Martín 137. Another biographer, Manuel Ortega, refers to 77 volumes of Pulido's Collected Works and more than 2000 medical articles (58). Pulido studied under Esquerdo in 1869–70 (64). Ortega and Pulido Martín provide hagiographic accounts of Pulido's very productive life.

32 The serialized article ran to seven instalments. To a modern reader the praise heaped on Esquerdo's institutions smacks of sycophancy, especially in view of the more modest assessments of Carabanchel by alienists visiting from abroad such as F.A. Jelly and Edward C. Seguin (1843–96) (381–84). Villasante and Huertas judge the article to have, "a hagiographic tone and an overblown style full of excesses," "un tono hagiográfico y un estilo muy barroco repleto de excesos" (30). Their article suggests that there may have been competition for patients amongst newly founded asylums at the time such that Esquerdo's loyal disciples may have had motives for praising his private institution at the expense of the government-financed Leganés. Pulido heaped contempt upon Leganés, with its undoubted underfunding and structural shortcomings, but saw fit to retract his criticism of the staff and the treatment of patients there once he had actually visited it. He does underline, however, the bad design of the institution and appeals for government resources to effect improvement. The correspondence in *El siglo médico* follows Pulido's criticism in, "Barcelona médica II" of 16th December 1888, the administrator, J. Del Mazo's protest, "Los manicomios de España" of 30th December, and Pulido's reply, "Los manicomios de España: El de santa Isabel de Leganés" of 17th February 1889.

1885 to study the development of Jaime Ferrán's vaccine against cholera[33] and, in the face of opposition of government and medical establishment circles, was his dogged champion.

Similarly distinguished was the Valencian, Luis Simarro (1851–1921). Briefly medical superintendent of the asylum of Leganés, where his attempts to make autopsies routine were frustrated by the religious directors, he studied psychiatry under Jean-Martin Charcot (1825–93) and Valentin Magnan (1833–1916), and anthropology under Paul Broca (1824–80) in Paris in 1880–85. He returned to Madrid in 1886 in time to testify in the defence of the insane priest, Cayetano Galeote, on trial for the murder of the bishop of Madrid. He was later appointed to the first chair of experimental psychology in Madrid. As a young man in 1867 he had the distinction of being expelled from a teaching position for holding Darwinian ideas, then under papal interdiction.[34] He is also remembered for having introduced into Spain Golgi's technique of staining nerve tissue with silver chromate. Once back in Madrid, he shared details of the method with Ramón y Cajal, who subsequently used them in his foundational investigations in neurohistology.[35]

Another contemporary was Jaime Vera (1859–1918) who is well-known as the co-founder with Pablo Iglesias of the Spanish Socialist Party, the PSOE (*Partido Socialista Obrero Español*), in 1879 and for his subsequent socialist writings. He began adult life, however, as a physician working as an *alienista*-disciple of Esquerdo and was employed for a time at Esquerdo's asylum at Carabanchel Alto. It was on the basis of his experience of patients with General Paralysis of the Insane (G.P.I.) seen at that asylum that he wrote a monograph on the disease in 1880 with a preface by his mentor.[36] He accompanied Ángel Pulido in a visit of inspection of the asylum of Leganés in 1888.

33 "Tras de la inoculación colerígena".
34 Vidal Parellada 23–24, Bandrés, Llavona and Campos 185.
35 Vidal Parellada 52, 83.
36 *Estudio clínico de la parálisis general de los enajenados*. Madrid: Moya y Plaza, 1880.

Other protégés of Esquerdo, who achieved prominence in professional life, listed by Ortega (65) are Rafael Salillas (1854–1923), criminal anthropologist who founded the *Revista General de Legislación y Jurisprudencia* in 1886, and who together with Luis Simarro, submitted draft legislation to Congress on asylums for the criminally insane; Victoriano Garrido an *alienista* who also worked at Carabanchel, whose interest in criminology is reflected in *La cárcel o el manicomio. Estudio médico legal sobre la locura* (1888); and finally José María Escuder (1853–1921) alienist, politician, writer and committed degenerationist who worked at the Carabanchel asylum for six years, and who collaborated with Simarro and Vera as expert defence witnesses in the trial of the Galeote in 1886, and of Martín Larios in 1888.[37] His two main books are *Quemas y crímenes* (1881) and *Locos y anómalos* (1895).

This group of highly talented *alienistas* owing loyalty to an influential teacher is strikingly reminiscent of the "circle of patronage" seen in France and described by Jan Goldstein.[38] This informal institution in France played a large part in establishing patterns of thought in psychiatry through disciples inspired by Philippe Pinel (1745–1826), Jean-Étienne Dominique Esquirol (1772–1840) and Bénédict Morel (1809–73). In Barcelona, the leading Spanish alienist of Galdós's day, the Catalán, Juan Giné y Partagas (1836–1903), inspired his own following. The Madrid "school" inspired by Esquerdo, if not actually working for him, shared his *alienista* belief in an organic basis underlying mental disease and the need for reform of care for the mentally ill in Spain.[39] This generation of brilliant *Young Turks* based

37 Vidal Parellada 49. Escuder was also an uncompromising evolutionist who saw religion and science as incompatible (Glick 270). Galdós attended the Galeote trial as a journalist and reported on it for *La Prensa* of Buenos Aires on 21 April and 9 October 1886.

38 *Console and Classify* chapter 4.

39 Villasante and Huertas draw attention to the minimal advances in the understanding of psychiatric disease that can be attributed to Esquerdo and to the dubious existence of any real Madrid "school" of alienism. In no way comparable to Pinel, Esquirol or Giné y Partagas, Esquerdo appears to have earned the leadership of his disciples more by his generosity of spirit, oratory and charisma. His entrepreneurial zeal in founding two private asylums may have had some bearing on the closeness of the group. Francos Rodriguez describes him as "an ardent, brilliant and colourful

in Madrid would have been in touch with each other and with the latest currents of medical thought. Whether or not they knew Galdós personally, they would all have known Tolosa Latour, and their knowledge would therefore have been at Galdós's disposal, if and when he wished to augment his own independent enquiries.

A memoir links Galdós with two of the leading surgeons of the time, Alejandro San Martín and Enrique Diego-Madrazo. Both are listed by Marañón as frequent guests at Galdós's home, together with Tolosa Latour (*Elogio* 145–46), and he recalls that in the Galdós home, "there was always a physician who possessed a magical authority."[40] In addition, Marañón records that even when he was only recently qualified as a doctor, Galdós held a striking admiration for his medical knowledge, "for him, from the beginning, my medical knowledge [inspired] a kind of devotion, as if before a superior power."[41]

Surrounded by such an illustrious group of physicians, it is not surprising that Galdós should have evinced such admiration for the profession. In this he was not alone, for physician-writers such as Pío Baroja and Gregorio Marañón recall the high social prestige of medical men of the time, even if that regard did not survive into the new century. The former writes, "The prestige of the modern physician is truly enormous. [The prestige of others] is nothing beside the admiration and devotion accorded to the

orator, and many hundreds of us gathered to hear him habitually ending the sessions with noisy displays of enthusiasm," "un orador fogoso, brillante, pintoresco, y a oírle acudimos muchas centenares de jóvenes que acabábamos todas las sesiones con sonoras muestras de entusiasmo" (Granjel, *Francos* 216). Esquerdo published in 1878 a series of lectures "Conferencias sobre enfermedades mentales" in *El Anfiteatro Anatómico Español* and, in parallel, in the *Revista de Medicina y Cirugía Práctica*. They are striking for their rhetorical oratory, name-dropping, and for the scarcity of original thought. They appeared in the year after Esquerdo had opened his private asylum at Carabanchel.

40 "siempre hubo en aquella casa un médico que tenía mágica autoridad" (*Elogio* 145).

41 "una suerte de devoción suya, como ante un poder superior, que para él lo eran mis conocimientos médicos, desde su incipiencia" (*Elogio* 145).

doctor, especially the young doctor."[42] Marañón emphasizes the importance of physicians in the view of political liberals of the day, "This prestige that the physicians had in the mind of the liberals of the nineteenth century was, to a certain extent, a preoccupation of the century."[43] He refers to "those doctors of the dramas of Galdós, surrounded by a mythical halo, who exercised an almost religious influence in the society of their time."[44] On the other hand, he cautions, "this problem of the brilliant physician, who appeared and achieved his greatest height in the last third of the nineteenth century, and now appears to be beginning a decline," and continues, "The literature of the period, that of Dudet (sic), Zola, Galdós and many others, contributed greatly to the elevation of the physician."[45] Marañón describes the rigours of medical training, "many years of difficult study, a hospital apprenticeship full of unpleasantness, and afterwards, almost always, the hard practice of the rural doctor or [that] of small urban communities. Because those who triumph are few." He continues, noting the rarely achieved social ambitions of many studying medicine for the wrong reasons, "They only aspire to pass like lightening through the academic stage and achieve the qualification in order to exchange it on the following day, as they suppose, for social triumph that, naturally, almost never follows."[46]

42 "El prestigio verdaderamente enorme de la época moderna es el del médico. [otros prestigios] no son nada al lado de la admiración, de la devoción que produce el médico, sobre todo el médico joven" (*Galería* 811).

43 "Era, en cierto modo, una preocupación del siglo, este prestigio que el galeno tuvo en la mente de los liberales del siglo XIX" (*Elogio* 145).

44 "aquellos doctores de los dramas de Galdós, rodeados de un halo mítico, que ejercieron en la sociedad de su tiempo una influencia casi religiosa" (*psiquiatras* 83).

45 "este problema del médico brillante, que apareció y alcanzó su apogeo en el siglo XIX, hacia su último tercio, y de ahora parece que comienza a declinar." [...] "La literatura de la época, con Dudet (sic), Zola, Galdós y otros muchos, contribuyó poderosamente a la magnificación del médico" (*Vocación* 335).

46 "muchos años de estudio penoso, un aprendizaje hospitalario lleno de sinsabores, y después, casi siempre, la áspera profesión del médico rural o de las sociedades urbanas modestas. Porque son muy pocos los triunfadores." "Aspiran solo a pasar como ralámpagos por la etapa académica y poseer el título para cambiarlo al día siguiente, suponen ellos, por el triunfo social que, naturalmente, no llega casi nunca" (*Vocación* 336).

A glance at the pages of the journal *El genio médico-chirúrgico* in the 1880s, when Galdós was writing many of his most memorable medical portraits, amply confirms Marañón's latter assessment. Letters to the editor from rural physicians complain of being at the mercy of the politically affiliated local bosses, *caciques*, dominant in local affairs and of the scant respect and unreliable remuneration that were returned for their labours. There was an ongoing debate on the extent to which doctors should emulate the abnegation of the priest in the practice of their profession. In a letter entitled *Un lamento de un rural*, a country doctor complains, "there will be few doctors who have not had to complain of serious quarrels in their districts with mayors' offices and the party bosses, who are their *lords* and *masters*."[47] The editor, himself, sizes up the situation:

> Only the doctor is obliged to work for free, to offer his unpaid services although they expose him to mortal [risk] attending the plague-ridden in a stinking and disgusting dwelling […] we [must] say that the doctor is the priest of science whose sacred responsibility he cannot betray although in every other way he may be a man as others and no one cares for his family, though it be numerous, when he leaves it poor and orphaned.[48]

The complaints include a report of exactly such a death of one doctor, Augustín Martín Niviero, who, having sent his family away to escape a cholera epidemic affecting the village of Gerindote in 1885, continued to treat his patients, only to fall victim to the disease himself and to die in his home unattended.[49] Given these conditions of rural practice, it is unsurprising that many doctors should wish to try their fortunes in Madrid.

47 "serán pocos los médicos que no tengan que lamentar sérios disgustos en sus partidos con los Ayuntamientos y los caciques, que son sus *dueños* y *señores*" (Barrios 214, author's italics).

48 "Sólo al médico es al que se le obliga á trabajar de balde, á prestar sus servicios gratuitos y aunque con ellos exponga también su vida asistiendo á un moribundo apestado en hedionda y repugnante morada […] es el médico, decimos, el sacerdote de la ciencia, á cuya sagrado carácter no le es posible faltar aunque en todo lo demás sea hombre como todos y nadie se cuide de su familia, si quier (sic) sea numerosa, cuando la deje pobre y huérfana" (Tejada y España, *Arte* 14).

49 "¡Pobres medicos rurales!" 456.

There, however, they encountered a different set of problems, not the least of which was fierce competition as a result of professional overcrowding. A review by the medical editor, Tejada y España, in 1881 found that an upper echelon of no more than thirty doctors attended to the needs of the aristocracy and the wealthy, leaving 200 to attend to patients belonging to the less highly paying beneficent societies that exercised collective bargaining to reduce professional fees. There remained a further 1300 doctors competing to provide medical services for a middle class of about 100,000, giving rise to, "need, struggle, and as a result of interminable pushing and shoving, scandals and disreputable behaviour." With the result that doctors experienced, "that well-being and ease they enjoyed in earlier times has been reduced to the unimaginable."[50] The numerous poor had nothing to contribute to doctors' incomes as they attended hospitals and clinics where medical services were provided without charge.

It appears that infighting and recrimination among physicians were common. In an editorial in 1881, a Dr Calatraveño laments, "those individuals who regard the profession as a source of profit, and not what it really is, a calling [...] within our house [of the profession] we have those who rob our honour; we are our own enemies." He goes on to decry, "the lack of collegiality and medical morals," and claims that, "if a united profession were a fact, we would soon see the disappearance of that gang of *curanderos*, witches and midwives that surrounds us."[51]

It appears that cut-throat professional competition in Madrid was not the only problem the profession had to cope with. From the very top of the profession, the secretary of the Royal Academy of Medicine, Matías Nieto Serrano, launched a stinging rebuke of the shortcomings of Spanish

50 "la necesidad, la lucha, y como consecuencia, esa interminable série de atropellos, escándalos, y bajezas," with the result that doctors saw, "reducido hasta lo inconcebible aquel bienestar y desahogo de que disfrutaba en otras épocas" (*profesión* 4–5).

51 "aquellos individuos que miran la profesión como un lucro, y no come lo que realmente es, un sacerdocio [...] Dentro de casa tenemos los que nos roban la honra; nosotros somos nuestros mismos enemigos". "[L]a falta de compañerismo y moral médica"; "Si la unión médica fuera un hecho, pronto veríamos desaparecer esa falange de *curanderos, brujas* y *comadres* que nos cerca ..." (666, author's italics).

medicine, both in the capital and the provinces. After stereotyping the German for his calm thoughtfulness, the Frenchman for his sense of beauty and the Englishman for the energy of his practical labour, he characterizes the Spaniard for his emotion added to empty, "experimental" prose. He ironically lambastes the lack of originality and productivity in Spanish medicine:

> Spanish medicine, always prudent and constrained in its flights of theory by respect for tradition, by the profound awareness of the limits imposed upon human reason, has not dazzled the world with proud systems [of thought], with dominating theories; it has not distinguished itself by analysis; it has not preferred to occupy itself in mastering Nature, chasing and dissecting it with wearisome perseverance. In contrast it has had the virtue of laborious study, of being aware of the folly of the metaphysical flights of fancy suggested by ambitious physics, and has placed a barrier against the mistakes that arise from excessive confidence in insufficiently studied data.[52]

Nieto Serrano was not alone, for in 1892 the distinguished surgeon and Galdós's friend, Alejandro San Martín, found it appropriate to end his conference at the *Ateneo* on medical advances coming from the Americas on a critical note. He laments the low numbers of Spanish doctors seeking advanced medical training in Paris, London and Berlin, in comparison with those visiting from Latin America. In addition, he adds his personal aspiration, "that the men of science who have made advances for us in demanding investigations as a result of the [medical] resources brought

52 "La Medicina española, prudente siempre y contenida en sus vuelos teóricos por el respeto á la tradición, por la profunda consciencia del límite impuesto á la razón humana, no ha deslumbrado al mundo con sistemas arrogantes, con doctrinas avasalladoras; no ha sobresalido en el análisis; no se ha ocupado preferentemente en dominar la Naturaleza, persiguiéndola y disecándola con fatigosa perseverancia. Pero en cambio, ha tenido la virtud de aprender asiduamente, de sentir la vanidad de los desvaríos metafísicos, sugeridos por un Física ambiciosa, y de poner un dique á los desaciertos que emanan de excesiva confianza de datos insuficientemente estudiados." (287) A striking example of the prolix rhetoric of the time is to be found in Ángel Pulido's "Conflictos entre la frenopatía y el código. Carta dirigida al Dr. Esquerdo" in the first volume of Guislain's *Lecciones orales* [...], in which he rivals Esquerdo in his talent for rhetorical verbosity.

from America, pardon our present backwardness."[53] It would appear that the medical profession had improved little by 1902 when Ángel Pulido, then Director General of Health, felt obliged to observe that the medical classes, "are backward classes," *son clases retrasadas* (*Sanidad* 78), and, "still remain in the first stages of professionalization, which it is urgent to speed up for the good of society and for the [medical] classes themselves."[54] He bases this judgement partly on the high prevalence of infectious diseases throughout the county, and especially on the "true disaster and huge shame," *verdadero desastre y una grandísima deshonra*, of 2000 deaths in Madrid in 1900–01 (11,685 in all of Spain) from smallpox, at a time when vaccination campaigns in other countries were making significant progress in eradicating the disease (22–24).

The development of the medical professions in Spain in the nineteenth century had been a difficult one. Attempts to regulate them had been frozen during the *Guerra de Independencia* and were subject to cycles of legislation and cancellation as Liberal administrations in Spain alternated with the absolutist regimes of Ferdinand VII.[55] Despite at least seven legislative attempts to standardize medical education and to establish fewer categories of medical practitioner, the situation remained chaotic. Ever since the appearance of the medical press in the 1840s, its assessment of the ills of the profession was uniformly depressing.[56] In 1862, the year that Galdós arrived in Madrid, a report appeared in *El siglo médico* in which

53 "á que los hombres de ciencia que nos han adelantado en las costosas investigaciones motivadas por las cosas venidas de América, disculpen nuestro actual atraso" (54).

54 "permanecen todavía en las primeras fases de una evolución professional, que urge acelerar para bien de la sociedad y de las clases mismas" (*Sanidad* 80).

55 The legislative see-saws, and the first attempt to rationalize medical practitioner's certification in 1827 are recounted by Albarracín, *Titulación* 18–29.

56 "Ever since the medical press appeared in [national] Spanish life, its diagnosis of the status of the physician in society is unanimous and monotonous: penury, disdain, carelessness, ungratefulness, oppresion, debasement, humilliation, scorn," "Desde que la prensa médica irrumpe en la vida española, su diagnóstico acerca de al situación del médico ante la sociedad es unánime y monocorde: pobreza, desprecio, desconsideración, desagradecimiento, opresión, envilecimiento, humillación, vilipendio" (Albarracín, *Professión* 305).

Francisco Méndez Álvaro summarized the variety of practitioners then treating the Spanish public. Many of them had limited training but were nevertheless able to compete with university-trained doctors for the fees of sick patients. Méndez lists, *ministrantes*, *facultativos de segunda clase*, *medico-cirujanos habilitados*, *practicantes*, *facultativos habilitados de segunda clases* and *cirujanos sangradores o de tercera clase* among the categories crowding the health care occupations. In all, Méndzez Álvaro counted no fewer than 35 distinct categories (*Fragmentos* 739). Twenty years before the correspondence on the plight of rural physicians already quoted, Méndez Álvaro describes them as, "dominated by capricious or brutal party bosses [...] who use qualified physicians as a pretext for infighting or to display their awful skills for malignant intrigues."[57]

The *Gloriosa Revolución* of 1868 resulted in two major changes in the credentialing of health-care practitioners. One was the legislation signed by Ruiz Zorilla that mandated a simplifed three-tier system of academic titles in medicine, those of *Bachiller*, *Licenciado* and *Doctor*. The second was freedom of teaching, *libertad de enseñanza*, which removed governmental control from the selection of professors and institutions that could prepare students for medical examinations.[58] This enabled competent teachers like the surgeon Federico Rubio and the *alienista* Esquerdo to give classes in a new atmosphere of academic freedom. The complete deregulation during the six years of the *sexenio liberal* (1868–74), however, resulted in the appearance of institutions of very variable quality springing up all over the country awarding their own degrees to hundreds of their own graduates with an associated collapse of academic standards.[59] In this academic

57 "dominada por caprichiosos ó brutales caciques [...] que suelen tomar á los facultativos titulares como pretexto para librarse duros combates ó para lucir su funesta habilidad en malignas intrigas" (*Fragmentos* 738).

58 These legislative changes are described in the installment of Sanson y Portillo's *La profesión médica en España* in *El siglo médico* of 17 Nov. 1878.

59 "the formation of medical societies to provide teaching [...] that awarded degrees to hundreds who joined those awarded [degrees] in official institutions, whose academic standards had disappeared completely," "la formación de sociedades médicas para dar enseñanza [...] que concedieron títulos a centenares, a los que venían a unirse los

free-for-all thousands of more lowly qualified surgeons were able to present themselves for examinations to upgrade to the new qualifications of *licenciado* or *doctorado* in Medicine and Surgery without giving any account of where or for how long they had studied (Sanson y Portillo *17 Nov. 1878*, 723). Similarly the number of candidates acquiring the new title of *practicante* doubled (723). The result was that the profession was flooded with practitioners who were not trained to the standard that their diplomas implied. In addition to them remained medical practitioners who had not upgraded their professional training or qualifications, but continued to practise in a dozen or more categories that had survived the reorganization of 1868 (Albarracín, *Titulación* 70).

A further complication of the post-*Gloriosa* freedom of teaching was that the right to issue professional diplomas was no longer under central governmental control, but was delegated to provincial degree-awarding institutions. This delegation was followed by a flood of hundreds of forged diplomas, increasing what had already been a chronic problem.[60] In the flood of revolutionary liberal fervour, some members of congress had even suggested in 1874 that in the free exercise of the professions, formal qualifications be abolished altogether (Carceda 70).

After the Restoration of the Bourbon monarchy in the person of Alfonso XII at the end of 1874 and the reassertion of central governmental authority, the *libertad de enseñanza* was abolished in the following year, and the award of a medical *Licenciado* restricted to those who had studied for at least five years (Carlan, *Revista* 625). In 1875, a committee was formed to suppress the industry of forged professional diplomas in order to restore public confidence, though an article in *El siglo médico* two years later suggested that it had achieved little (Carlan, *Nombramientos* 17).

---

obtenidos en los establecimientos oficiales, cuyo rigor había desaparecido totalmente" (Albarracín, *Titulación* 63).

60 "Los títulos falsos." *El siglo médico* 22 Aug. 1875. 543. Sanson y Portillo records that in 1874 several members of the faculty of medicine of the Central University of Madrid were expelled for fraud in the conduct of professional examinations (*17 Nov. 1878*, 274).

Writers to *El siglo médico* suggested that despite the attempted rationalization of the profession after the Revolution of 1868, many of the profession's problems remained. Just before the Restoration, Ramón Vezalde complains that practitioners were still being authorized to practise medicine after only two years' training. He repeats the complaint that doctors find themselves obliged to testify on forensic cases without remuneration and that, should they die while treating an epidemic, the law guaranteeing a pension to their widows is not being implemented (657–58). In addition to this he finds the profession largely responsible for its own predicament because of its failure to act collectively:

> At present the conviction that asking for even a slight remedy of the professional problems that have afflicted us as of old makes little sense [...] it is rooted profoundly in the self-same medical class. This is borne out with sad eloquence by the fact that a meeting of the Medical-Pharaceutical Association could not even be convened for a forthcoming day.[61]

He observes that physicians are filling prescriptions and marketing cures of dubious merit while pharmacists undertake medical consultations, and all in competition with, "the plague of healers and charlatans."[62]

The problems of practitioners of all stripes providing services which they were not legally entitled to give, *intrusismo*, stirred up bitterness among health care professional throughout the nineteenth century. Two Royal Decrees attempting to limit such practices in 1894 and 1898 are eloquent testimony to the fact that *intrusismo* remained "an unsolved plague at the end of the nineteenth century,"[63] A second plague, for which the professions themselves were responsible, arose when practitioners, even when fully qualified, yielded to the pressure of competition for paying patients

61 "El convencimiento de que en la actualidad es pretensión poco sensata la de solicitar ni aun leve remedio á los males profesionales que de antiguo nos afligen [...] se halla arraigado profundamente en la clase médica misma, como con triste elocuencia lo está acreditando el hecho de que no poderse siquiera la Asamblea de la *Asociación Médico-Farmacéutica*, convocada para un día próxima" (659).

62 "la plaga de curanderos y charlatanes" (658).

63 "una lepra sin solución a fines del siglo XIX" (Albarracín, *Intrusos* 334).

by marketing themselves, and medications of doubtful value, to the general public in newspapers and posters. Such charlatanism was rife in both cities and in rural areas. A third variety of medical fraudster, the *secretista*, offered a range of secret powders, elixirs and other miraculous medications that were claimed to remedy all known ills. Finally the traditional folk healer, the *curandero*, thrived particularly in rural areas, among the illiterate and the gullible and might call upon a variety of spells and incantations in his or her work. At mid-century, spiritualism and animal magnetism were much in vogue (Albarracín, *Intrusos* 357). A consequence of this tribe of "healers" was that the reputably trained physician had to cope not only with competition, legitimate and otherwise, from his professional peers but also these usually untrained practitioners, who might have loyal followings in the communities where the physician practised.

So in spite of stronger central governance and the return of relative stability after the Restoration of 1874, an improvement in the status of the medical profession remained illusory:

> In sanitary and medical enforcement, every year we are a little worse. Our administration exhibits indifference, complete indifference in the face of the dangers that charlatanism poses to society [...] in addition we suffer the insult of a goodly number of physicians and not a few pharmacists, violating all respect for morals, who busy themselves shamelessly chasing miserable small change, behaving like ridiculous clowns letting down their class, and dishonouring the universities where they received their scientific education and their academic credentials.[64]

Even after the abolition of *libertadad de enseñanza*, there remained ten medical schools, the free institutions that had arisen in Salamanca, Sevilla

64 "En policía *sanitaria* y *médica*, cada año estamos un poco peor. Nuestra administración se mantiene indiferente, completamente indiferente, en medio de los peligros con que el charlatanismo amenaza a la sociedad [...] sufrimos además la afrenta de que buen número de médicos y no escaso de farmacéuticos, rompiendo con todos los respetos a la moral, corren impúdicos en busca de un poco de mísero cobre, convertidos en ridículos botargas injuriando a la clase, y deshonrando las universidades en que recibieron su educación científica y sus grados académicos" (Carlan, *Año* 2, author's italics).

and Zaragoza having been regularized by the central government. Their standards of teaching were very variable. Sanson y Portillo estimates that three good institutions would have been enough to provide for the needs of the 16 million Spaniards then populating the country. He attributes the legitimization of unsatisfactory schools to local deal-making and self-interest, and as a result, the descent upon the public of hundreds of poorly trained practitioners (*24 Nov. 1878* 739).

Repeated criticism in the medical press over the years suggests that medical health professionals in Spain were inherently incapable of setting aside personal issues for the greater good of the profession. As early as 1849, an editorial complained of, "… the apathy, the indifference or despondency that rules the majority of medical men when they see time pass without any improvement in their unhappy situation […] the lack of unity among doctors, their rivalries and their poorly disguised envy."[65] Almost 30 years later Vezalde sounded the same notes in reaction to the incapacity of Spanish medical men to organize for their mutual benefit, "… a spirit so clearly opposed to all associations […] No one believes in anything; no one trusts anyone; doubt, indifference and disastrous selfishness have almost dissolved any social [links] […] envy, rivalries, insaciable ambition, the most exaggerated self-importance and ruinous egoism disrupt and poison everything …"[66] Only in 1889, could a writer concede that, in spite of Spain's backwardness and the absence of adequate governmental support for public health, the lot of the profession had improved, "It's true that our Spain is relatively backward […] that public health does not receive the support to which it

65 "… la apatía, la indiferencia o desaliento que de la mayoría de los profesores se apodera al ver que pasan los años sin que se remedie su triste situación […] la desunión de los profesores entre sí, sus mutual rivaldades y sus mal disimuladas envidias" ("*M.D.*" 25).

66 "… un espiritu tan claramente adverso a toda asociación […] Nadie cree en nada; nadie confía en nadie; la duda, la indiferencia y el funesto personalismo, tienen casi disuelta la sociedad […] las envidias y las rivaldades, las ambiciones insciables, el amor propio más exagerado y el ruin egoísmo lo perturban y los envenenan todo …" (*¡Meditamos!* 69).

has an undeniable right, that our class is bitter about many abuses ...; but despite all this, however, we are increasing a little in prestige."[67]

The contrast that university-trained physicians sought to draw between themselves and unauthorized practitioners undoubtedly included a desire to affirm their professional status, expensively acquired at the more reputable institutions. This, in turn, invites consideration of the nature of the medical education that took so much time and money. What was the academic background that distinguished the university-trained physician from the rival *intrusos*, *charlatanes*, *secretistas* and *curanderos*, with whom they had to compete?

A vivid account of medical education from 1887–94 is that of Pío Baroja. He details his experience in a series of autobiographical reminiscences, many of which also formed the basis for his novel, *El árbol de la ciencia*, published in 1911. Baroja had decided upon a career in medicine in early adolescence and began a course of premedical studies in 1887 at the age of fourteen. His studies included physics, general chemistry, mineralogy and botany, and zoology and were taught at the Institute of San Isidro in Madrid. He quickly passed the examinations of the courses with the exception of the chemistry which, to his surprise, he passed soon afterwards. Baroja's introduction to medical studies, however, was not propitious. He had been expecting firm discipline in the lectures and was appalled to encounter a raucous atmosphere in which students applauded a pathetic old professor who appeared not to realize that he was being made fun of.

In his second course, which was taught at the medical school of San Carlos in 1888–89, Baroja began medical subjects proper and began anatomical dissection. His classes were entitled, Descriptive Anatomy and Embryology, Histology, and Technical Anatomy. He passed all three classes on the second attempt. In his third medical course, the second year at San Carlos, Baroja studied more Anatomy and Embryology, a second course

67 "Es verdad que nuestra España está relativamente atrasada [...] que la salubridad pública no logra aquella protección a que tiene incontestable derecho, que nuestra clase se resiente de muchos males ...; pero sin embargo, de todo esto algo vamos ganando en prestigio" (*Año nuevo* 3).

of Anatomical Techniques, Physiology, and Personal Hygiene. Though uninspired by the professors, Baroja managed to pass all four. The fourth year of 1890–91 saw Baroja meet two influential professors with whom he clashed temperamentally. The first was José Letamendi, who taught Pathology, and who Baroja considered had a "certain literary talent but none as a man of science," dismissing his lectures as, "all verbal fireworks and wordplay."[68] Letamendi did, however, stimulate Baroja to read Kant, Fichte and Schopenhauer, the last of whom he found particularly rewarding. More serious were Baroja's confrontations with Benito Hernando, professor of therapeutics, whose personal attacks partly based on his antipathy toward Baroja and his fellow Basques were, *arbitrario, caprichoso e insoportable* (*Medicina* 589). According to his own account, Baroja, was unwilling to be cowed by Hernando's petty rudeness and answered him in kind, which incensed the professor to the point that he told Baroja that he should continue his medical studies at another university (589). Hernando backed up his recommendation by seeing to it that Baroja failed twice in his examinations of Pathology and Therapeutics, despite his being been well-prepared for them. As a result, he continued his studies at the medical school in Valencia, reflecting that he had known many bad-tempered professors (589).

Apart from classes, Baroja's fourth year in Madrid (his third medical year) was one in which he began to attend the wards of the *Hospital General*, which was to have a profound influence on his attitude to the profession. He saw for instance, drugs from the hospital being sold by staff to the pharmacies of *calle Atocha*, and groups of card players and gamblers about the hospital itself (593). His impression of the nursing sisters, *las Hermanas de la Caridad*, was that they seemed primarily preoccupied with administrative matters and with calling for a confessor when a patient's condition was critical (594). Baroja's experience of clinical medicine took a still grimmer turn when he attended Madrid's hospital for venereal diseases,

68 "cierto talento literario pero nada de hombre de ciencia" (*Medicina* 587); "todo palabrería y fuegos artificiales" (*Medicina* 588).

San Juan de Dios, which he likened to a cross between a hospital and a lunatic asylum (596).

There he found women terribly debased by prostitution in a filthy, evil-smelling room where they were treated by a sadistic old man, doctor Cerezo, who punished patients with isolation and a diet of bread and water, when rules were infringed. Baroja unforgettably describes in his memoir (*Medicina* 597) and in his novel (*Árbol* 83), the instance of a pathetic patient seeking consolation in a pet cat, which Cerezo orders to be hunted down and killed. Near to hitting the old man for his brutality, Baroja is restrained by a friend, but resolves never again to return to the hospital. It has since been observed that this brutalizing experience of *San Juan de Dios* and the behaviour of despotic professors toward him as an impressionable 18 year-old had a long-term effect on Baroja, and was at the root of the radical pessimism of his writing.[69]

At the medical school Valencia, Baroja failed General Pathology for a third time, but claims that he then learned the art of "studying mechanically," after which he passed all his examinations. In his fifth year (his first in Valencia) in 1891–92, he passed Therapeutics and Pathological Anatomy and by the end of the year had finally passed General Pathology, Surgical Pathology and Medical Pathology together with Paediatrics. In the sixth year of his training (1892–93), Baroja passed Obstetrics and Gynaecology, Topographical Anatomy, Operative Medicine and the first classes of Clinical Surgery and Clinical Medicine. In the seventh year, at the age of 21, he took a class in Public Hygiene, Legal Medicine and Toxicology and

69 "It is clear that the young Pío at his 18 years, cannot bear the sadism of the doctor Cerezo, nor the behaviour of other despotic professors who he encounters in his career, and that this [...] led him to a radical pessimism that, to a certain extent, lies in all his work," "Es evidente que el joven Pío con sus dieciocho años, no puede suportar el sadismo del doctor Cerezo, ni las actitudes de otros despóticos profesores que encuentra en su carrera, y eso [...] le llevan a un radical pesimismo, del que, en cierta manera, está impregnada toda su obra" (Cabezas 32). Another well-known physician who was forced to transfer to a different medical school for expressing opinions that the teaching faculty did not like was Luis Simarro (Vidal Parellada 29). In his case the transfer was from Valencia to Madrid.

finished his academic requirements with second classes in Clinical Surgery, and Clinical Medicine.

With classwork behind him, Baroja presented himself for the examination of *licenciatura*. He passed the first, theoretical part easily and, upon advancing to the practical, second part, was advised by the examiner that he needed more clinical experience. While realizing that his 5–6 months of clinical experience were truly not adequate, Baroja insisted on continuing with the rest of the examination, which involved a case of gangrene that he claimed "anyone could have diagnosed." For the third part of the practical examination he was asked to identify and isolate the subclavian artery in the body of a cadaver. Despite the examiner's reservations about the extent of his practical experience, he passed the examination (*Medicina* 605) and was awarded the *licenciatura* in medicine by the University of Valencia on 19th October 1893.

Baroja immediately returned to Madrid to study for the degree of *doctorado*, but found the teaching there dull. The courses included History of Medicine, Anthropology, Public Hygiene and Epidemiology, and Chemical Analysis. The only entertaining professor was one who regaled them with reminiscences of his exploits in the National Militia. Only at this point did he attend ward rounds with Jacobo López Elizagaray in the General Hospital and begin to learn a little about auscultation [of the chest] and about the technique of percussion to identify the margins of a [usually abdominal] mass (607).[70] Having completed his course work for the *doctorado*, he then wrote a thesis on "Pain," which he dismissed as being completely unoriginal. On discussing his thesis with the three examining professors of the doctoral tribunal, they gave him the impression of not having read it. After a humorous interchange with one of them, the surgeon Alejandro San Martín, he left with his title of doctor, "knowing very

70 This is a striking admission on Baroja's part and gives some idea of the predominance of theory in his teaching for the *licenciatura*. Good medical teaching in more recent years has students beginning to learn the basic skills of the clinical examination, which include auscultation and percussion, at the very beginning of their clinical training.

little or almost nothing of real medicine, like the majority of students."[71] He was 21 at the time.

Writing 16 years after his graduation in medicine, Baroja's view of his medical professors and the methods of instruction remained critical. He lambasted the custom of dividing classes into groups with the result that only a third or a half received instruction on each subject:

> The professors of medicine had an approach that could not have been more stupid. In the universities where I studied, subjects were taught incompletely. Something ridiculous in any profession, but even more ridiculous in medicine. In Medical Pathology, one shift of students studied infections, another group nervous diseases; another only the diseases of the respiratory tract. Doing this can only be explained in the context of a Spanish professor, who is generally the quintessence of superficiality.[72]

His memories of his professors were indeed bleak, "I do not remember any professor who knew how to teach, who managed to communicate enthusiasm to those he taught and who had any understanding of the mind of the student."[73] Baroja is known for his acerbic criticism of those he did not like (Guimón 111), however, and his comments might be discounted, were it not for the fact that a very similar account of medical teachers comes from Comenge:

> teachers who only care about their salary and rank, about their private patients and the accumulation of distinctions; not about teaching, for which they were like a

71 "sabiendo muy poco o casi nada de Medicina verdadera, como la mayoría de los estudiantes" (*Medicina* 613).

72 "Los profesores de Medicina tenían un criterio tan estúpido que no cabe más. En las Universidades donde yo cursé, las asignaturas se cursaban a medias. Cosa ridícula en cualquier profesión, pero más ridícula aún en Medicina. Una tanda de médicos había estudiado en Patología Médica las infecciones; otra tanda las enfermedades nerviosas; otra, sólo las enfermedades del aparato respiratorio. No se explica más que en un profesor español, que generalmente es la quinta esencia de vacuidad, el hacer esto" (*Estudiante* 197).

73 "Yo no recuerdo de ningún profesor que supiera enseñar, que llegara a comunicar afición a los que enseñaba y que tuviera alguna comprensión del espíritu del estudiante" (*Estudiante* 197).

> kind of oyster stuck to a text of anatomy, pathology or therapeutics that they never abandoned or revised in teaching [their] courses, [worn out] has-beens who fought against the scientific.[74]

Referring to medical teaching in the first half of the century, Comenge declares that ecclesiastical domination of medical education had condemned it to outmoded scholastic tradition, "ecclesiastical influence distorted medical education, separating it from the experimental sciences in order to confine it to the prolonged and almost sterile study of dead languages and outdated texts."[75] He notes that academic studies in preparation for a career in medicine were identical to those undertaken by those destined for the law and the priesthood. The latter, perceiving more opportunities in the lay world after the liberal revolution of 1868, defected from the church in large numbers to reassign themselves to medical training, taking advantage of lax requirements in provincial teaching institutions as a result of the *libertad de enseñanza*. The medical profession consequently became overcrowded with poorly trained individuals, many with an indifferent commitment to their new vocation, bringing with them a rigidity of mental outlook associated with their original career choice (372).

Finally, a testimony to the faithfulness of Baroja's depictions comes from his fellow-physician, Gregorio Marañón, who, on welcoming him to the *Real Academia Española* in 1935, praised his books for their, "exact and fundamental documentation of the Spain of our time – or, at least, of an aspect of our Spain [...] it is very much in his dialogues where he achieves

74 "maestros que solo se cuidaron de la nómina, del escalafón, de la particular clientela y de acumular distinciones; no de la enseñanza, de la que fueron una suerte de ostras pegadas á un texto de anatomía, patología ó terapéutica que no abandonaron ni reformaron jamás, explicando, muchos cursos, antigallas que pugnaban con el estado de la ciencia" (414).

75 "la eficacia eclesiástica torció la educación médica, separándola de las ciencias experimentales para enfrascar en el dilatado estudio y casi estéril de las lenguas muertas y caducos textos" (371).

his great precision and reality [in] the human and genuine version that he gives us in his books."[76]

With training behind him, Baroja practised medicine for the next year in the small Basque town of Cestona, which at that time had a population of 2,470.[77] He gives an account of that period, the only one in which he actually practised as a doctor, again both in his autobiographical memoirs and in the fictionalized account in *El árbol de la ciencia*. His account includes stories of horseback rides at night to make emergency calls to distant patients in the snows of winter, or in driving rain. In addition, it was his duty to perform post-mortem examinations on any local people who appeared to have died violently. He felt ill-prepared for the work and sensed that his diagnostic skills were inadequate, an awareness sharpened by the fact that his inexperience seemed to be apparent to the villagers about him:

> The position of village physician then was, and continues to be now, difficult, poorly paid and extremely responsible. To me it seemed distressing and hard, although it certainly had its compensations.
>
> I did not have a bad reputation as a doctor. My old landlord, Vishente, the husband of the lady sacristan, used to say of me: "Yes, he has knowledge; but *practical* [experience] is what he *lacks*."[78]

Superimposed upon these harsh circumstances were difficulties with other medical professionals of the town. His introduction to the author-Jesuit priest, Padre Coloma, got off on the wrong foot when his professional rival introduced him as being a "revolutionary" (*Aristocratismo* 959). Worse

76 "una documentación más exacta y fundamental de la España de nuestro tiempo – o, al menos, de un aspect de nuestra España [...] la versión humana, genuina, que nos da en sus libros es justamente en el díalogo donde alcanza su mayor precisión y realidad" (*Contestación* 321–22).

77 Cabezas 44.

78 "El oficio de médico de aldea era entonces, y seguirá siendo ahora, difícil, mal pagado y de gran responsabilidad. A mí me parecía penoso y duro, aunque ciertamente, tenía algunas compensaciones.

No tenía mala fama como médico. Mi antiguo patrón, Vishente, el marido de Dolores *la Sacristana*, decía de mí: '– Sí, ya sabe; pero la *frática* es lo que le *palta*'" (*Médico* 624, author's italics).

still, the same physician attacked him for seeing one of his patients in an emergency when the physician himself was away from the village and, even more, for suggesting referral of the seriously ill patient to a specialist in San Sebastián. The grounds for this complaint appeared to be that such a referral would reduce the number of house visits for which the rival physician would be able to charge. All this was too much for Baroja, who gave in his notice after a year. He later wrote elsewhere in his memoirs, "In the practice of rural medicine, one sees very extraordinary, at times, terrible things, which give an impression, perhaps too vivid a one, of the selfish and brutal nature of man."[79] He never practised medicine again.

Baroja's account of rural, medical practice might be considered to be jaundiced if it did not correspond closely with the complaints aired in the early 1880s in the pages of *El genio médico-chirúrgico*, in the recurring criticisms of Sanson y Padilla in *El siglo médico*, and with the warning of Marañón. Furthermore, the accuracy of Baroja as a witness of the social conditions of the poor of his time and of Madrid's infrastructure has been studied by Carmen del Moral Ruiz, who finds his descriptions to tally closely with other accounts of the period.[80]

This being so, it seems all the more extraordinary that Galdós, with his genius for accurate social description and his interest in clinical conditions, should say so little about the critical state of the Spanish medical profession. While the Madrid focus of his contemporary novels would have given him little motive for studying the conditions of rural doctors, one might have expected at least a hint of the difficulties that city doctors endured. But it appears that the struggle for professional survival of Madrid physicians and their competition with charlatans and *curanderos* receives no mention in his novels. Instead idealized, infinitely caring and wise physicians usually

79 "En la práctica de la Medicina, en la aldea, se ven cosas muy extrañas, a veces terribles, que dan una impresión quizá demasiado viva del fondo de egoísmo y de brutalidad del hombre" (*Recuerdos* 678).

80 del Moral finds Baroja's account of the poor in Madrid very accurate, but comments that he devotes little space to the upper and upper-middle classes. She finds him less reliable in his descriptions of working-class political movements, notably socialism (193–95).

occupy the foreground. There are occasional references to inept physicians in the novels, but they are usually not identified by name. Galdós unleashes bitter criticism of doctors in his press articles, with their squabbling over rival theories on the nature of cholera and their collective failure to limit the spread of the disease and, again, physicians remain unidentified. This may possibly have been a matter of prudence since journalists at the time could find themselves challenged to a duel if the subject of criticism considered his honour to be offended.[81]

Whether Galdós chose to disregard the endemic problems of the medical profession of his time in his novels, or simply saw them as irrelevant to his art is not evident. He clearly had a passion for medicine and revered the members of the medical elite who became his friends. Physicians appear in his novels with a greater frequency than in the work of any other contemporary novelist, usually appearing in a positive light. Granjel finds more than 50 medical characters, prompting him to refer to the *Colegio médico galdosiano* (*Médico* 167).[82] What is abundantly clear is that Galdós possessed a singularly penetrating mind that enabled him to master many more contemporary medical ideas than have been recognized.

Descriptions of medical conditions are so widely distributed in Galdós's writing that this study can offer no pretence of completeness. Emphasis is given to the characters that suggest borrowings from medical sources that were available to Galdós or to his medical friends. The latter, being part of

81 As late as 1900 the offices of *La correspondencia de España* had a fencing room with a French fencing master for the instruction of its employees, "The profession of journalism is exposed to affairs of honour and one must know how to handle the sword and the sabre in case it comes to a duel," "La profesión de periodista está expuesta a los lances de honor y hay que saber manejar la espada y el sable por si llega el caso de batirse" (Cansinos-Asséns in Mateos Fernández 333). Ángel Pulido's son records that his father took up fencing specifically to defend himself against people whose feelings and material interests might be threatened as a result of Pulido's vigorous journalistic involvement in controversial issues. The son records that Pulido's aggressive sparring partner was none other than his fellow-disciple of Esquerdo, the hot-headed Valencian Escuder (Pulido Martín 41).

82 This number appears to be exceeded only by Pío Baroja in whose work approximately 200 physicians appear (Guimón 108).

Madrid's elite, were accustomed to travel to conferences and medical centres in France, Germany and England as an essential part of their professional lives. Their linguistic abilities were such that many were able to study texts in the original languages; their cumulative knowledge would have represented a major resource for Galdós. With this in mind, there is considerable reliance upon French medical texts, which were highly influential in Spain at the time. Comenge comments on this dominance, "the invasion of foreign texts in their own language or translated into Spanish was considerable; one could say that our peninsula became a splendid market for the French, and in this way our [medical] science was dependent on the foreigner."[83] The half-French Tolosa Latour was an agent of this cultural hegemony by virtue of his knowledge of French medicine and through his translations into Spanish of French medical texts. Where possible, an attempt has been made to rely upon contemporary medical texts, avoiding anachronistic analysis of medical ideas in Galdós's novels in the light of later developments. This is especially so in the context of his portrayal of insanity and mental aberration, which were penned before Freud's theories became widely known. This is in accordance with Galdós's professed lack of enthusiasm for psychodynamic theories, as it was recalled by Marañón.[84]

83 "la invasión de escritos medicos fué más considerable en lengua primaria y traducidos al castellano; diríase que nuestra península se convertió en mercado espléndido de los franceses, y, así nuestra ciencia siguió un feudo del extranjero" (413).

84 "the new era in the art of the novel that was coming, under the influence of Freudianism, with which don Benito never had any concern," "la nueva era que advenía en el mundo del arte novelesco, bajo los auspicios de freudismo, con el cual don Benito no tuvo nunca nada que ver" (*Elogio* 145).

CHAPTER 2

Epidemics: Cholera, Influenza and Smallpox

Like the inhabitant of any other large city in the nineteenth century Galdós was very well aware of epidemics. These outbreaks of disease in unusual numbers were most often derived from infections that at other times maintained a continuous, lower profile in the community (endemic disease). They were subject to recrudescence as a result of local factors such as bad weather or hunger that lowered the population's resistance to disease. Diseases often followed poor harvests when bread became more expensive and beyond the reach of many of the unemployed. Diphtheria, scarlet fever and measles were present throughout the year but sometimes attained epidemic proportions during cold winter months. Smallpox was never absent from Madrid but, for a variety of reasons, it achieved epidemic proportions in 1890.

The second, less common, form of infection and death in unusual numbers arose when an infecting organism spread outside its traditional geographic range to affect populations previously unexposed to it. The example of this in Europe, *par excellence*, was cholera, the disease responsible for the majority of Galdós's medically related articles in the press during the years that he wrote for *La Nación* (1865–66, 1868) and for *La Prensa* of Buenos Aires (1884–1894). In the latter articles, medical topics appear more frequently than any other scientific subject (Shoemaker, *Estudio* 23). Galdós not only witnessed the cholera epidemics of 1865 and 1884–85 in Madrid firsthand, but in June 1885 was able to interview someone who had the perspective of having lived through the four epidemics to strike Madrid, and who had vivid memories of fleeing those of 1833–34, 1855 and 1865.[1]

1 Pérez Galdós, Benito. *Obras Inéditas: Crónicon (1883–1886)*. vol. 6. Madrid: Renacimiento, 1924. 194. Hereafter referred to as *Ghir VI*.

While cholera had long been endemic in India, its first recorded eruption outside the region of the River Ganges was in 1817. Its spread into Europe in the nineteenth century has been attributed to increasing trade with India, the movement of large colonial armies about that subcontinent, and an increasing number of pilgrims making the *Haj* to Mecca.[2] After the first pandemic, which spread from Bengal to involve China and Indonesia in 1816–1826 but remained within Asia, the second international pandemic reached Russia, Western Europe and the United States, causing hundreds of thousands of deaths between 1829 and 1851. It reached Spain in 1833 through the port of Vigo and resulted in a national death toll of about 300,000, of whom nearly 5,300 were in Madrid.[3] Gripped by superstitious fear engendered by the epidemic in 1834, a Madrid mob attacked a number of convents and slaughtered friars who they believed to be spreading the contagion by poisoning wells.[4] The third pandemic of 1852–60 spread throughout Asia and the Americas with its major impact in Russia where there were over a million deaths. It was during the course of this epidemic that John Snow's study of the epidemiological pattern of infection in the London district of Soho led him to elucidate the role of faecally contaminated drinking water in the spread of the disease. Though Snow, like everyone else at the time, was ignorant of the bacterial cause of cholera, his work resulted in the celebrated removal of the handle of the Broad Street pump which ended local spread of the disease.[5] In that pandemic, cholera arrived in Spain by sea and was first recognized in Vigo and Barcelona. In

2 Fernández 166; Hauser (*cólera* 399). Medical knowledge of cholera in 1885 and its history in Spain is summarized in Hauser's article and book on the epidemic that was coloured by his adherence to Pettenkofer's *telluric* theory. This theory postulated that special conditions of the soil needed to be present before the bacillus caused disease. Much of Galdós's writing corresponds closely with Hauser's account. Another contemporary account is that of the demographer, Jimeno Agiús, who describes the disproportionate vulnerability of infants under a year of age and of women of reproductive age (*cólera*, 22).

3 Fernández, *Repercusiones* 138.

4 Hauser, *Madrid* 294–95. Galdós includes a fictional account of these events in his *Episodio Nacional, Un faccioso más y algunos frailes menos*.

5 Snow 44–47.

its peak years of 1854–55, it resulted in over 236,000 deaths in the entire country, with 4,210 of them occurring in Madrid.[6] Sanitary precautions that were instituted included quarantine, *cordones sanitarios* and disinfection, but they were soon found to be ineffective in preventing spread of the disease. The fourth pandemic of 1863–75 mostly struck Europe and Africa and is memorable in medical history partly for the action of William Farr in London where, taking advantage of Snow's work, he identified, and put a stop to, a supply of contaminated water with the result that he was able to abort a local outbreak.[7] Cholera had its greatest impact in Spain in 1865, coinciding with a period of falling population associated with economic crisis, emigration, and political instability that led to the calling of elections.[8] Appearing first in Valencia, it was carried throughout the country by people fleeing to the north to escape the disease. In Madrid, as was customary, the epidemic was most lethal in the poorly fed and abysmally housed families of the city's poorest districts. Dislocation of the workplace and interruption of the distribution of food left many day labourers unable to feed their families, reducing their resistance to disease still further. The mortality in Madrid was reported as being just under 2,900, while that in the nation as a whole was 119,000,[9] though contemporary reports such as that of Varela de Montes suggest that the authorities concealed the true scale of the 1865 epidemic.[10]

In 1865–68 Galdós wrote a total of 130 articles for *La Nación* mostly concerned with cultural affairs, musical reviews, art criticism and politics, but in a few of them he also describes the cholera epidemic of 1865. In that August, he refers to the spread of the epidemic from Alexandria in Egypt and Ancona in Italy and comments on the association of deaths with local flooding. He describes the epidemic as an "exterminating angel" and a "wandering Jew," and records that it fills cemeteries as it passes. In addition he takes the neo-Catholics to task for interpreting the epidemic as a

6 Fernández, *Repercusiones* 138.

7 Eyler 119–20.

8 Fernández, *Epidemias* 99, 95.

9 Fernández, *Repercusiones* 138.

10 Varela de Montes 5.

divinely ordained punishment for Spain's support of the heroes of Italy's unification. Galdós ironically comments that:

> In addition, some frightened folk say that cholera has arrived in Madrid without permission, and there is no shortage of people who claim to have seen it, increasing to the number of four the victims affected this week; but the neighbours of this supremely healthy capital can remain calm. They are all lies; cholera isn't in Madrid and is not thinking of coming for a long time, assured that we quietly enjoy the lashes of innumerable plagues and public calamities, quite as fearsome as those that the pestilential visitor from India carries in his pocket.[11]

An article follows in September again asserting that there is no significant cholera in Madrid, but advising his readers to avoid fruit and vegetables that are not in season. He also recommends avoidance of disquieting emotions of hypochondria and strong feelings, which might predispose to infection, and advocates the fumigation of homes with sulphur.[12]

11 "También dicen algunos asustados que el cólera se ha metido sin pedir permiso en Madrid, y no falta quien afirma haberle visto, y eleva al número de cuatro las víctimas que han inmolado en esta semana; pero ya pueden estar tranquilos los vecinos de esta salubérrima capital. Todo es mentira; el cólera no está en Madrid ni piensa venir en luengos tiempos, seguro de que disfrutamos mansamente el azote de innumerables plagas y calamidades públicas, tan temibles como las que trae en el bolsillo el pestilente viajero de la India" (*Nación* 118).

12 *Nación* 140–41. Hauser records that in the epidemic of 1833, medical authorities banned over- and under-ripe fruit in the belief that they were unhealthy and predisposed people to abdominal disorders (*Madrid* 292). Conflicting opinions on the dangers of fruit and vegetables were aired during the 1833 epidemic in the *London Medical Gazette*, "Do vegetables produce cholera?" (261–64). In John Sutherland's 1850 report on cholera in Britain in 1848–49, an outbreak affecting the crew of a ship carrying a cargo of fruit to Hull was attributed to the crew's excessive consumption of plums (9–10). The belief that cheerfulness was a preventative against cholera was longstanding, illustrated by Corbyn's advice as a result of his experience of cholera in India (100–02). Galdós echoes this belief in the importance of mental attitude in *Un faccioso más ...* where he has Gracián dismiss traditional remedies in favour of, "The best antidote against the sickness was [...] courage and disdain for the infection itself," "El mejor antídoto contra el mal era, [...] el valor y el desprecio del mal mismo" (270).

This relatively light-hearted account of the disease is followed in October by a more sombre reference to victims of the "terrible traveller of the Ganges."[13] Despite his account of the sound of hammering of coffin lids, he notes hopefully that funeral processions are becoming less common, suggesting that the number of cholera deaths may be diminishing. He speculates further that the applications of sulphur and phenol may have had a salutary effect, combined with the influence of a frigid wind from the north-east then blowing through Madrid. Galdós's serious tone continues as he again takes the neo-Catholics to task for suggesting that cholera deaths are God's punishment for Spain's proposed recognition of the newly unified Italian state, with its associated curtailment of papal secular power. He also notes the frequency of traditional religious processions and public prayers to beg relief from the epidemic, and suggests that they may be counter-productive by giving rise to panic, "which is a second epidemic more devastating than that which afflicted us on Sunday and Monday."[14] He returns to these themes in December in his review of the year, entitled, "The Seven Plagues of 1865," more specifically identifying an outbreak of panic that accompanied the epidemic.[15]

The last great outbreak of cholera in Spain of 1884–85 arrived in August through the port of Alicante rapidly extending to Valencia and defying attempts at quarantine and the burning of infected persons' clothes. As was often observed, the epidemic subsided during cold winter weather only to break out again in the warmth of the following spring, when it extended throughout the country in the summer of 1885. Migrant farmworkers

13 *Nación* 169.

14 "Una segunda epidemia, mas asoladora que la que nos azotó el domingo y el lunes" (*Nación* 170).

15 The power of panic to predispose to cholera endorsed by Galdós was widely held at the time though, like everything else about the disease, it was subject to disagreement. Varela is sure that, "fear saves more victims than courage" having seen both the brave and the timid swept away, and reasons that the fearful are likely to take more precautions to avoid the contagion (6). For Varela, religious processions, "instil confidence and tranquilize the spirit of the believer" (8).

travelling to northern parts of the country in search of work were identified as vectors.[16]

While Galdós's account of the 1865 cholera outbreak in Madrid had been that of a relatively inexperienced reporter, the 1885 epidemic found him at the height of his powers and able to do justice not only to the political, social and economic turmoil, but also to the medical complexities of the epidemic. In addition, this epidemic was much better recorded, with better statistics and wider coverage in the press, than earlier visitations of the "son of the Ganges." To some extent this was the result of more relaxed rules of press censorship. The national mortality of over 120,000, of which 1,366 were accounted for by deaths in Madrid,[17] was associated with a lower mortality in the capital than previous epidemics. This was attributed to the inauguration after 1855 of a relatively clean water supply from the río Lozoya via the canal of Isabel II, the installation of a network of 120 km. of sewers, and the relief of some of the worst crowding by demolition of the old defensive walls of the city.[18] However, the epidemic provoked bitter, polarizing and destabilizing political argument. The Minister of the Interior, Romero Robledo, adhered rigidly to the traditional sanitary measures of *cordones sanitarios* and quarantine, even when it was abuntantly clear that they failed to limit spread of the disease and served only to disrupt commerce and the supply of food to cities. This, together with his intransingent opposition to inoculation against the disease, contributed to his resignation from the Cánovas government in July 1885 (Fernándes Sanz 381–82).

In his letters to *La Prensa* of Buenos Aires, Galdós often writes about the social and economic dislocation resulting from the epidemic and of the fear that it inspired, believing that fear of the disease, in itself, predisposed to the infection.[19] As the disease approached Spain in July 1884, he voices

16 Hauser, *Madrid II* 306.

17 Fernández, *Repercusiones* 138.

18 Hauser, *Madrid II* 314. Hauser attributes the reduced mortality to the evacuation of the most crowded dwellings in the poor lower suburbs, the *barrios bajos*, and the disinfection of dwellings where cholera appeared (306).

19 Fernández, *Epidemias* 149, notes the contemporary belief that fear predisposed to contracting cholera. Galdós appears to have subscribed to this view as the evil

the widespread suspicion that official measures to prevent it from crossing frontiers were a waste of time, likening their effectiveness to the ability of cobwebs to stop a cannon ball:[20]

> The recognition of the uselessness of sanitary measures at ports is becoming widespread since they have no purpose other than to annoy travellers and harass commerce and to extract from both sizable sums of money designed to feed a swarm of doctors[21] who would have nothing to do without official jobs in isolation hospitals and sanitary boards.[22]

By November of 1884 the number of cases in Alicante and Barcelona appeared to be diminishing with the cooler weather, only to recur in an unexpected outbreak in Paris:

> With the alarm has arrived that medical-administrative calamity christened *sanitary precautions*. These seem to be the invention of the physicians immortalized by Molière, for whom the great poet had a dislike that he could not and would not disguise. Isolation facilities at sea and on land are already installed with their humiliations and abuse.[23]

---

consequences of fear and panic recur in his descriptions of the epidemics (*Ghir. VI*, 185, 218, 227, 233), and conversely, his suggestions that equanimity and cheerfulness are protective (*Ghir. VI*, 255, 265).

20 *Ghir. VI* 179.

21 In contrast with the idealized portrayals of individual doctors in his novels, Galdós seems to have had no difficulty in criticizing anonymous members of the profession as a group. He had ample scope for this in his descriptions of dithering, ineffectual and opportunistic doctors that recur throughout the course of the 1884–85 epidemic (*Ghir. VI*, 27, 29, 35–53, 74, 179).

22 "Va cundiendo la idea de la inutilidad de las medidas sanitarias en los puertos pues, generalmente, parecen no tener más objeto que molestar a los pasajeros, vejar al comercio y extraer de aquéllos y de éste fuertes sumas destinadas a dar de comer a una multitud de médicos que no tendrían nada que hacer si no existieran las plazas oficiales en los lazaretos y Juntas de sanidad" (*Ghir. VI* 24).

23 "Con la alarma ha venido también esa calamidad médico-administrativa a que se da el nombre de *precauciones sanitarias*. Éstas parecen invención de aquellos médicos inmortalizados por Molière y a los cuales tenía el gran poeta una malquerencia que no podía ni quería disimular. Los lazaretos marítimos y terrestres están ya instalados con sus vejámenes y atropellos" (*Ghir. VI* 74, author's italics). The extent to which

Galdós does not hide his exasperation at what appears to be self-serving doctors gathering fees for services of questionable value at the same time that they squabble unproductively about the nature of the approaching contagion. This open dissention was due to the fact that the profession was divided as to whether cholera was or was not an illness that could be caught directly from an infected person. On the one hand, the *Anticontagionists* pointed to medical attendants in close contact with cholera victims who did not contract the disease and theorized that distant spread, such as through foul, miasmatic air would circumvent patient isolation. In contrast, the *Contagionists* observed that the diarrhoea of patients could be dangerously infectious and that isolation and disinfection of victims was necessary to prevent spread of the disease:

> the arguments between doctors here renew the confusion of past days. There is a so-called "Health Council" in which the Contagionists and Anticontagionists war daily in such a fruitless fashion that it would be better if they all went home. As the causes of the epidemic remain a mystery, everything that is said there serves to increase the uproar and worsen the situation.[24]

---

the citizenry loathed disinfection and the assaults of the disinfectors is indicated by Hauser who records that, in order to avoid them, madrileños would hide cholera deaths from the authorities and consult a folk healer, *curandero*, in preference to a trained physician (*Madrid II* 308).

24 "[…] aquí las discusiones entre médicos renuevan la confusión de los días pasados. Hay un Consejo que llaman de Sanidad en el cual los contagionistas y los anticontagionistas dan una batalla cada día, tan sin fruto, que más valdría que se fueran a sus casas. Siendo aún un misterio las causas de la infección epidémica, todo lo que allí se dice sirve para aumentar el barullo y empeorar la situación" (*Ghir. VI* 74). Indecision over the contagionist/anticontagionist debate was not confined to physicians in Spain, since many European governments enacted and then relaxed their quarantine legislation in the course of the nineteenth century (Ackerknecht, *Anticontagionism* 587). Ackerknecht, himself, admits that, given the information then available, he would have had, "a very hard time" in deciding between the two explanatory theories, concluding that, "especially economic outlook and political loyalties will determine the decision" (589). The miasmatic theory goes back to classical times and held that disease is spread by foul air, the word *malaria* being derived from it (Latin: *mala*=bad, *aria*=air). In a select committee report before the House of Lords in 1846, Edwin Chadwick had summarized it thus: "all smell is, if it be

As the epidemic took hold of the country in 1885, the ineffective sanitary measures of Romero Robledo, "whose sanitary campaign has been the butt of endless cutting jokes and satires,"[25] were reversed. This led to a farcical situation in which the government changed course but was unable to persuade citizens to stop isolating and fumigating hapless travellers. The results of local attempts at contagion control could be cruel in the extreme, as Galdós notes with biting humour:

> The government thunders against isolation units and orders their disappearance in vain. Either [the villagers] do not obey or pretend to do so while returning to the routine shortly afterwards. In some villages the "isolation hospital" is a tumbledown hay barn, an unused mill, a cattle yard or something similar, where there are no beds or food or any kind of comfort or the necessities of existence [...] "isolation facilities" are roofed by the open sky so that the detained can enjoy the delights of dew at night and the midsummer sun by day ...[26]

---

intense, immediate acute disease; and eventually we may say that, by depressing the system and rendering it susceptible to the action of other causes, all smell is disease" (109). Even after 1884 and Koch's discovery by of the bacillus responsible for cholera, leading figures in public health such as Edwin Chadwick, Florence Nightingale and Max von Pettenkofer continued to subscribe to the miasmatic theory into the 1890s.

25 "cuyas campaña sanitarias han sido objeto de picantes burlas y de sátiras sin fin" (*Ghir VI* 208).

26 "En vano el Gobierno truena contra los lazaretos y dispone su desaparición. O no le obedecen, o fingen obedecerle para volver al poco tiempo a las andadas. Llaman lazaretos en algunos pueblos a un destartalado pajar, un molino sin uso, un corral de ganado o cosa parecida, donde no hay camas ni alimento, ni comodidades de ninguna clase, ni aun lo más necesario para la existencia [...] Hay lazaretos que tienen por techumbre la bóveda del cielo, para que puedan los detenidos disfrutar las delicias del relente por las noches y un sol canicular durante el día ..." (*Ghir. VI* 251–52) Galdós's recurring condemnation of sanitary precautions was part of a growing intolerance of bureaucracy, particularly on the part of those of liberal political sympathies. Sanitary precautions were based on the principle that cholera was contagious. Ackerknecht notes that, "Contagionism would, through its association with the old bureaucratic powers, be suspect to all liberals, trying to reduce state interference to a minimum" (*Anticontagionism* 567).

Galdós's interest in the epidemic went well beyond its socioeconomic dislocation as he delves into the epidemiological data then available. In July of 1885, he observes that while the current outbreak seemed to be less serious than those of 1833, 1855 and 1865, it was again most severe among the poorly fed and badly housed unfortunates who lived near swampy ground, where they were also subject to malaria.[27] He returns to this association in his letter of July 1885 where he describes the severe outbreak in Aranjuez with its extensive open water fed by the rivers Jarama and Tajo,[28] and the epidemics in the extensively irrigated fields of Valencia and Murcia.[29] He notes, in contrast, the relative sparing of arid areas such as Cartagena and Alicante.

Galdós wrote his accounts after the identification of the cholera bacillus by Koch in 1884 when the role of micro-organisms in epidemic disease was becoming increasingly apparent, and refers to, "millions and millions of microscopic organisms."[30] However, Koch's organism was but one of several claimed to be responsible for cholera at the time and his announcement was far from universally accepted. In this state of uncertainty, therefore, it is unsurprising that the vocabulary of bacteriology should coexist with that of the traditional miasmatic theory, "a great development of organic miasmas."[31] It was still widely believed that bad smells, in and of themselves, could transmit disease and this remained a basic tenet of anticontagionist belief that survived to the end of the century. In the poorly cleaned and drained streets of most cities of the time with their rotting organic material of all kinds, the concept of miasma was an unavoidable one in dealing with contemporary reality.

Galdós expresses popular impatience with the inability of doctors to agree on the basic nature of cholera and blackly jests:

27 *Ghir. VI* 216–17.
28 *Ghir. VI* 236.
29 *Ghir. VI* 238.
30 *Ghir. VI* 239.
31 "una gran elaboración de miasmas orgánicos" (*Ghir. VI* 238).

> if [the microbe] comes while they are trying out this or that system against it, it will decimate our population and when it leaves, weary of so much havoc, two equally sad things will remain: a mountain of cadavers and another mountain of booklets on cholera pathology. God spare us the double attacks of the epidemic and medical pedantry![32]

In answer to a eugenic "medical eminence," who maintains that cholera is a valuable means of weeding out sickly and unfit members of society, Galdós prays to God that the epidemic not come, and that they are relieved of the doctors who argue all they want [with] such contradictory opinions about the manner of curing it.[33]

For all his humorous impatience with medical disagreements, Galdós took the trouble to inform his readers about the facts of the disease as they were then established. He quotes the medical consensus that the microbe of cholera is spread by the faeces of its victims, especially in a humid environment associated with open water.[34] He mentions the likelihood that some madrileños, unemployed and suffering from disrupted food supplies, are dying not of cholera but from hunger.[35] He quotes the inconclusive debate between Letamendi and José Olavide about the capacity of various chemical agents to destroy the cholera bacillus, with Letamendi improbably maintaining that the bacillus was impervious even to *aqua regis*, the highly corrosive mixture of nitric and hydrochloric acids.[36]

Galdós's critical sense of humour found a target not only in vacuous politicians and ineffectual doctors but also in the superstition and credulity to which communities were prone under the stress of the epidemic.

32 "si viene [tal microbio] mientras se ensaya contra él este o el otro sistema, diezmará nuestras poblaciones, y cuando se marche, fatigado de tantos estragos, nos quedarán dos cosas igualmente lastimosas: un montón de cadáveres y otro montón de folletos sobre patología colérica. Aparte Dios de nosotros el doble azote de la epidemia y de la pedantería médica" (*Ghir VI* 27).

33 *Ghir. VI* 29.

34 *Ghir. VI* 26.

35 *Ghir. VI* 197.

36 The inconclusive debate was reported by Galdós under the title of, "Un duelo científico" (*Ghir VI* 35–53).

He recounts the entertaining story of a carter who believed himself saved from cholera by the miraculous intervention of the Virgin of Puig through the application to his body of oil from the lamp at her shrine. Word of the miraculous cure spread widely in the province giving rise to pilgrimages of faithful folk in search of anointment with the supposedly miraculous oil. Galdós sagely adds that, "religious superstition has always played a large role in public disasters."[37] His black humour has its *denouement* in a following letter that June when he reveals that the sacristan selling the precious oil had died suddenly from a fulminating attack of cholera. Galdós archly surmises that the sacristan, himself, may have had no faith in the remedy that he was administering to folk coming from all parts of Valencia. More farcically still, he reports that the local cardinal-archbishop later opened an enquiry into the activities of the parish priest with a view to finding out what had happened to all the money paid by pilgrims in return for anointment with the oil.

One of the most serious and divisive issues that Galdós reports in the 1885 epidemic concerns the Catalán physician, Jaime Ferrán, whose development of an anti-cholera vaccine split the country into equally passionate supporters and opponents of his treatment. Gregorio Marañón later referred to Ferrán as "a unique instance in our history: a man of science who was argued about by people to the point of violence."[38]

Born in Tarragona in 1852 and trained in medicine at the University of Barcelona, Ferrán entered medical practice in Tortosa, but was keenly interested in bacteriology and followed Pasteur's discoveries closely.[39] His part-time study became all-consuming and was successful to the extent

37 "La superstición religiosa hace siempre un gran papel en todas las calamidades públicas" (*Ghir. VI* 192). In *Un faccioso más y algunos frailes menos*, Galdós vividly evokes the credulity of ignorant people frightened by the cholera epidemic of 1833 when he has them interpret supposedly holy soil imported by friars as poison for the entire population, designed to rid them of the Liberals (295–96). This erupts into a riot in which a mob led by Tablas murders Gracián and his fellow clerics in their convent.

38 "un caso único en nuestra historia: un hombre de ciencia que se discutió hasta la violencia por las gentes" (*Ferrán* 859).

39 I owe this description to the accounts of Bornside, Faus Sevilla and Fernández Sanz.

that a report of his work won a prize awarded by the *Real Academia de Medicina de Madrid* in 1884.[40] He developed an interest in the possibility of immunization against cholera, encouraged by the successful development of inoculation against fowl cholera (a different organism from the cholera of humans) and bacterial carbuncle of livestock (*bacera)* by veterinarians in France. Ferrán was a member of the team sent to Marseilles to study an outbreak of cholera there, and set up a small laboratory to study the bacillus. On his return to Spain, he succeeded in immunizing guinea pigs against the disease by injecting them with live cultures of the attenuated bacillus and proceeded to immunize himself with the same technique. In March 1885 he announced his findings to the *Real Academia de Medicina de Barcelona*, where the epidemic was beginning to take hold, and received a favourable response that was mirrored in the press. In the same month, he submitted a report to the *Académie des Sciences de Paris* which, for its own reasons, omitted to acknowledge having received it.[41] Feeling that he had made a sufficient public announcement of his discovery, Ferrán set up a makeshift laboratory in Valencia to produce the vaccine and was given permission to start his first large-scale immunization campaign in the town of Alcira.

His development of the vaccine had occurred too rapidly for conservative members of the medical profession, however. Some of them were not convinced that among all the other organisms found in the excretions of cholera patients, Koch's *Bacillus vírgula* (now known as *Vibrio cholerae*) was the one truly responsible for the disease. Though Koch's work had been published in Spain in the 1884, the year that followed saw many in Madrid's *Real Academia de Medicina* who were still discussing old ideas about the influence of atmospheric factors in the production of cholera epidemics.[42] Members of the *Academia* had not only not discussed Koch's discovery, which appeared tardily in *El siglo médico* in 1884,[43] but in the following year, when the cholera epidemic was at its height, demonstrated

40 *Memoria sobre el parasitismo microbiano* (Fernández Sanz 107).

41 Fernández Sanz 112.

42 Fernández Sanz 101.

43 Carlan. "Conferencia del Dr. Koch."

their sense of urgency about of the disease by occupying themselves exclusively with the consideration of syphilis.[44] Significant opposition to Ferrán developed in Madrid where a doctor Mendoza of the hospital of *San Juan de Dios* had the ear of the Minister of the Interior, Romero Robledo. From this time onwards, the anti-cholera immunization programme divided Spain on political and social lines with many older physicians and political conservatives condemning Ferrán's work as experimental and unproven, while mostly younger physicians and liberals hailed him as a champion of Spanish science and a saviour of the Valencian people. The violence and bitterness of the debate were often fuelled by the protagonists' ignorance of bacteriology and the nascent science of immunology.

Even among the medically well-informed, however, a number of distinguished physicians had reservations about Ferran's vaccine. Luis Simarro and Ramón y Cajal were both unconvinced, while Hauser, in his detailed analyisis of the 1884–85 epidemic published in 1887, complains that Ferrán's account of morphological variations in the *vírgula* comma bacillus had not be validated by others. He charges, in addition, that Ferrán's statistics were not freely available for inspection and that the dangers of vaccination with the broth of the supposedly attenuated germ were real, implying that the

44 Fernández Sanz recounts how Ángel Pulido returned from Valencia to give a talk on 30th April 1885 about Ferrán's anti-cholera vaccine at the Royal Academy of Medicine, which was met by complete lack of interest on the part of its members. The latter proceeded, instead, to continue with their speculations about syphilis (133). Luis Comenge, who also knew Ferrán and who was in the thick of the debate over his vaccine later commented on the Royal Academies of the time, "what is certain is that, with time, [the Academies of Medicine] changed into theoretical discussion groups, into honourable clubs, medical conversational forums, with very little influence on the life and welfare of [their] institutions," "lo cierto es que, con el tiempo, se trocaron en congresillos teóricos, en centros honorables, tertulias médicas, con muy escaso influjo en la vida y prosperidad de la institución" (396). In contrast, seven lively debates took place in the Madrid *Ateneo* in July 1885, in which a number of well-known figures, including Luis Simarro, argued against the safety of the vaccine (Fernández Sanz 128).

vaccine was not of sufficiently proven efficacy to warrant its use in a mass vaccination programme (*Estudios* 321–30).[45]

Such was the situation when Galdós penned a series of articles for *La Prensa* trying to make sense of the national uproar that was inflamed by conflicting reports on the safety and effectiveness of Ferrán's invention. Allowing for Galdós's natural sympathy for the liberal camp and his dislike of Romero Robledo, what emerges is a remarkably balanced account. The articles of June 1885 immediately proclaim the importance of Ferrán's work as an alternative to the patently ineffective isolation hospitals, quarantine and *cordones sanitarios* promoted by the government.

Galdós refers to the success of inoculations against smallpox promoted by Jenner, and against rabies developed by Pasteur, and attributes to Ferrán the discovery that *Bacillus vírgula* can be attenuated by changing the temperature and chemical conditions in which it is cultured. He describes the confidence with which Ferrán and his collaborators inoculated themselves following successful experiments in guinea pigs. He mentions the temporary discomfort of "benign cholera" that followed the injections, and the protection afforded against the virulent disease even in the unhealthiest environments. He writes, "the fact of immunity of vaccinated subjects seems indubitable. Those who receive the cholera microbe attenuated in culture have not been infected,"[46] but qualifies this by explaining that the duration of the immunity acquired after immunization remains unknown.

45 It should be added that established scientists who were removed from the inflamed environment of Spanish politics also had reservations about Koch's identification of *Bacillus vírgula* as a cause of cholera. The prominent British zoologist, E. Ray Lankester, wrote an article for the Pall Mall Gazette in October 1884 questioning Koch's methodology, while Koch's work was stoutly defended in a following issue by Julius Althaus. Lankester's criticism appears in translation in *El siglo medico* in February 1885, together with a report of Koch's published answers to criticism of his bacteriological conclusions. It is thus clear that heated debate was not confined to Spain.

46 "Parece indudable que la inmunidad de los vacunados es un hecho. Los que se asimilaron el virus colerígeno atenuado por el cultivo, no han sido atacados" (*Ghir. VI* 182).

In presenting immunization against cholera as an established fact, Galdós considers its theoretical basis, listing three possible explanations to account for its effectiveness: that the responsible organism loses its vital impetus in the human body, that the prophylactic organism consumes all the nutrients in the body required by an attacking organism, and that the prophylactic organism promotes the production of substances that kill it (*Ghir. VI* 183–84). Medical science would have to wait until the following decade for the correctness of the last explanation to be established.

Galdós addresses the opposition to Ferrán, which he notes is strong in official circles where the clique of the Minister of the Interior is hostile towards him. He notes that pending the findings of a scientific commission, Ferrán is to be allowed to continue with his inoculation programme (13 June) and, in the following month (4th July), that the [first] commission's report was so favourable that the threat of a ban on inoculation had been removed. He again expresses the opinion, which was widely held at the time, that fear of the disease predisposed people to it and notes that, "the faith of the inoculated destroys one of the principle agents of the disease, which is fear, and has to promote the success of the programme."[47]

His laudatory articles follow with a biographical sketch of Ferrán. This is followed by an account of the opponents of inoculation who claim that the proceedure is as bad as the disease itself, and who voice fear that numerous inoculations against diseases will be too much for the human constitution to tolerate. English and German critics, he writes, claim that administration of attenuated organisms destroys the vigour of the human race and makes it more vulnerable to disease and death. Galdós admits that he does not know if these arguments are valid but notes that they bring the logic of common sense to the debate. However, he also adds shrewdly that he doubts if common sense isolated from facts is sufficient to answer these questions, essential though it is in informing the quest for truth.[48]

47 "La fe de los inoculados, destruyendo uno de los principales agentes del mal, que es el miedo, ha de influir favorablemente en el éxito del sistema" (*Ghir. VI* 185).

48 *Ghir. VI* 190.

By the end of July, Galdós enthusiastically praises Ferrán, "among the benefactors of humanity, none is greater than this humble country practitioner [...] who has solved the greatest medical problem of modern times."[49] At the same time, however, he details the mounting forces of opposition that had arrayed against Ferrán, from the Minister of the Interior downwards, noting the prohibition, then permission, and final banning of the immunization campaign.[50] Contributing to this was Ferrán's disastrous encounter with the leader of a French commission of enquiry, led by one Dr. Brouardel, whose inspection, Galdós suggests, was superficial and biased. He avers that similar reservations about Brouardel's harsh criticisms were voiced in the French and English press (*Ghir. VI* 245–46).

The final ban of Ferrán's programme coincided with a spontaneous decline in the number of cholera cases, so that inoculation ceased to be front-page news. It was thus left to other researchers to confirm the effectiveness of his vaccine with less public attention and in a less fraught atmosphere.[51] As Galdós's account suggests, the Ferrán controversy threatened social cohesion in Spain and exposed antagonisms and fault-lines within

49 "No habrá entre los bienhechores de la humanidad ninguno más grande que este humilde médico de partido que [...] has resuelto el más colosal problema médico de los tiempos modernos" (*Prensa* 156).

50 Romero Robledo's opposition to Ferrán appears to have been based upon his obsession with traditional sanitary precautions and upon a personal dislike and suspicion of Ferrán. Fernández Sanz suggests that any possibility of compromise was finally extinguished when Romero was attacked by his political opponent, Castelar, who vigorously supported Ferrán (126). Having received the favourable report of the first commission sent from Madrid, government authorities then sent a second commission of enquiry staffed by less qualified people who produced an unfavourable report, which was clearly what they preferred to hear (Fernández Sanz 143–45).

51 Foremost among these was Pasteur's protégé, the Ukrainian Nikolay Gamaleya (1859–1940), whose announcement of prophylactic inoculation against cholera with an attenuated live strain of *Vibrio* was announced in 1888, followed by the development of an inoculation using the killed organism. Both of these advances had been made by Ferrán beforehand though, according to Bornside (532), neither Pasteur nor Gamaleya acknowledged this when the latter's work was announced.

its society, features of cholera epidemics that have been observed in other countries and at other times.[52]

Throughout his discussion of this terrifying epidemic, Galdós avoids being strident, as he condemns the worst government failures, and contrives to inject humour and sound common sense into his descriptions of events. As an illustration, in August 1885, he describes the fondness for religious processions in local communities, particularly those dedicated to the patron saint of plagues, San Roque. In one instance, he describes an expensively opulent, candle-lit procession that was "interminable" and wonders if some of the money spent might not have been well-employed in removing some of the accumulated filth from the streets, and cleaning the foul-smelling sewers that drained districts of crowded, miserable hovels (*Ghir. VI* 266). He concludes that "he is sure that San Roque himself would be pleased to be taken in procession through well-swept streets and not past filthy, stinking drains."[53]

No other epidemic in Madrid elicited from Galdós an account as long, or as detailed, as that of cholera of 1884–85. In 1889–90, however, there followed what Fernández has called, "the year of three epidemics"[54] in which a severe outbreak of influenza was followed by widespread smallpox, with a combined mortality of 6000, exceeding even the deaths in Madrid from the most deadly cholera epidemic of 1833. Increasing public anxiety further, cholera briefly reappeard, though in nothing like the numbers of 1885. The reduced number of its victims was probably due, at least in part, to residual immunity acquired by the Madrid population as a result of the epidemic of four years earlier.[55]

52 Morris 17, McGrew 1, Durey 1.

53 "Tengo la seguridad de que al mismo San Roque le ha de gustar que lo paseen por las calles bien barridas y no por albañales inmundos y mal olientes" (*Ghir. VI* 267).

54 *Epidemias* 209.

55 Fernández, *Epidemias* 243. Hauser records that it was as late as 1887 before a belated and complete overhaul of Madrid's antiquated and ineffective system of public sewers was at last begun. This improvement may have contributed to the limited impact of cholera in 1890. Even when he wrote in 1902, however, the majority of houses were still not adequately connected with the main sewers and lacked running water to

The most lethal of the three epidemics of 1890, influenza, was the subject of a long account by Galdós. In January of that year, he writes of the epidemic in Madrid from which he suffered himself, and from which numerous well-known people died.[56] He reports that initial attempts to dismiss influenza humorously have been replaced by a sombre seriousness as the disease extended not only to Spain but throughout Europe.[57] He observes that, unlike the case of cholera, a higher incidence of influenza is not seen in in damp regions since it appeared to afflict its victims in wet and dry zones equally. This undermined the rumour then prevailent that dry, cold weather was to blame. Galdós's interest in the epidemiology of influenza appears piqued partly by its sporadic outbreaks, without the geographic localization seen in cholera. Also in contrast with cholera was the observation that the well-to-do appared to suffer more from influenza than the poor. Galdós speculates that the wealthy may be more vulnerable to being chilled when they leave their dwellings, as a result of their homes being heated and more comfortable than those of the poor, the latter being more accustomed to the cold. Prefacing his comments by noting the lack of clarity and variation in medical explanations then prevalent, he describes a *Micrococcus grippe* as the responsible organism, reassuring his readers that it is much more benign than the microbes responsible for tuberculosis, diphtheria, typhus and cholera (*Ghir. VII* 229).[58] What follows is an interesting reflection by Galdós, "But one cannot rely on the benignancy of *Micrococcus grippe* because it is subject to the law of evolution like all organisms, [and] may very well rise from its modest category to that of

flush lavatories. Many dwellings continued to rely upon private cesspits, *pozos negros* (*Madrid I* 26).

56 *Prensa* 332.

57 Pérez Galdós, Benito. *Obras Inéditas: Crónicon (1886–1890)*. vol. 7, ord. y prólog. Alberto Ghiraldo, Madrid: Renacimiento, undated, 225, hereafter cited as *Ghir. VII*.

58 Influenza is now attributed to viruses, a class of microbe that had yet to be identified in 1890, though a sub-microscopic agent responsible for diseases like rabies was suspected. Many bacteria including *micrococci* are found in the secretions of patients with viral influenza. It is now surmised that it was superinfection with a bacterial pneumonia that most often killed the victims of influenza epidemics (Morens, Taubenberger and Fauci).

Estaphilococcus pyogono (sic), the microbe of pneumonia, and from there to adopt the terrible behaviour of the tubercle bacillus discovered by Kock (sic).[59] This speculation entertains the possibility that, just as the disease-producing characteristics of a microbe could be attenuated, as Ferrán had achieved in the preparation of his vaccine, so it was conceivable that a reverse process of increasing pathogenicity could evolve.[60] Galdós pursues this concept, recalling that many tuberculous patients have suffered from persistent catarrh and pneumonia, rather implying that the tuberculous process may have arisen from a chest infection caused by a more benign organism (230).[61] Also in relation to tuberculosis, Galdós reiterates the accepted wisdom of his time that the disease is the result of an inherited predisposition, an, "inability to resist the attacks of the terrible microbe."[62]

Returning to the influenza epidemic, Galdós observes that the attribution of infection to climatic conditions is difficult to reconcile with the varying severity of the disease suffered by people enduring the same weather. He concludes that a sudden chill on passing from a warm room

59 "Pero no hay que fiarse de la benignidad del *micrococcus grippe*, porque hallándose sujeto, como todo organismo, a la ley de la evolución, puede muy bien ascender desde su modesta categoría a la de *estaphilococcus pyogono* (sic), que es el microbio de la pulmonía, y de aquí pasar al empleo inmediato, o sea a desempeñar las terribles funciones del *bacilus* de la tuberculosis, descubierto por Kock" (sic) (*Ghir. VII* 229–30, author's italics).

60 *Pathogenicity*: capacity to cause disease. We are now familiar with the idea of bacteria becoming more dangerous as a result of becoming resistant to antibiotics. The concept of a microbe changing its character, and specifically its form, in a life cycle, particularly in the context of tuberculosis, was one that Ferrán favoured. Bornside comments that, "the idea of life cycles in the tubercle bacillus was investigated for the next fifty years before it was finally refuted" (518).

61 The nineteenth century witnessed much confusion in distinguishing between disease entities that we would now consider as being entirely different. In his doctoral thesis of 1884, for instance, Ramón Gómez Ferrer (1862–1924), cites received wisdom that syphilis in a parent might be manifest as scrofula in the child and that diabetes in a parent might result in tuberculosis in the child (Gómez *179*, 341). Francos Rodríguez quotes the conjecture that syphilis might be able to, "degenerate" into gout, rheumatism, tuberculosis and carcinoma (29).

62 *Ghir. VII* 230, also Lloréns y Gallard 13.

to the cold outside is unhealthy, as is wearing too many or too few clothes, finally concluding that behind it all is the phenomenon of individual *predisposición*, "the causes of which are very complex and difficult to resolve" (230–31). Only in November is he able to report that the epidemic is clearly in decline. This he attributes to a decrease in fear, associated with neighbourly provision of food and shelter for the vulnerable poor since, "the epidemic principally affects the hungry and barely clothed, and charitable associations achieve marvels."[63]

Taking a broader view of the social consequences of the epidemic, he observes collapse of the Christmas trade with resulting gloom, suggesting as causes that many are too ill to eat and are disinclined to exchange seasonal gifts. Galdós yet again returns to the theme that he voices repeatedly in connection with cholera epidemics, that is, the influence of people's mood on their vulnerability to infection, "fear began to disturb spirits and exaggerate the danger, producing the alarms typical of every epidemic."[64]

He notes that influenza does not have a fulminating form, like cholera, that can kill in a matter of hours, but observes that the daily death rate in Madrid still stands at 200 and is three times what would ordinarily be seen in one of Madrid's bitterly cold Decembers. He finally suggests that many deaths are not due to influenza alone, so much as to the bronchitis and pneumonia that complicate the disease.

Galdós appears not to mention the third epidemic, that of smallpox, that was contributing to the mortality among madrileños in 1890. Hauser would later attribute that outbreak to failure of the authorities to implement adequate vaccination programmes to forestall what was a preventable disease,[65] while Comenge, in contrast, attributes the not infrequent

63 "la epidemia se ceba principalmente en los hambrientos y desnudos, y las asociaciones de socorros hacen prodigios" (*Prensa* 384).

64 "empezó el miedo a perturbar los ánimos y a exagerar el peligro, y se han producido las alarmas propias de todo período epidémico" (*Ghir. VII* 233).

65 *Madrid II* 48–49. In London, by contrast, more energetic preventative measures resulted in a steady decline of smallpox victims and deaths after 1885 (Hardy 112). Monmeneu also laments the low vaccination rate in Madrid that he attributes to, "laziness or ignorance" (92), comparing it with the much lower rates of infection in

local outbreaks of smallpox more widely to the, "traditional negligence of the citizens."[66]

Galdós briefly mentions cholera again in 1890 in the context of localized outbreaks in eastern parts of the country, which not only did not spread, but were also accompanied by very few cases in Madrid. He again criticizes the, "inhumane, counterproductive and brutal" sanitary precautions being implemented at the frontier by the Portuguese, which completely interrupted communication between the two countries both by land and by sea, and which he relates to out-moded practices of the Middle Ages.[67] A final reference to cholera occurs two years later, when he notes recurrence of the disease in the Middle East and Russia, with extension to Northern Europe and, specifically, to Hamburg. In relation to that city, he observes that the lakes and open water of the adjacent Elbe delta predispose to cholera and adds the *telluric* narrative still current, "given its excessive moisture the soil of the city must predispose to the spread of epidemic cholera."[68] He records no victims in Spain then.[69]

In the course of two major and one minor cholera epidemics that Galdós witnessed in the course of his first 27 years in Madrid, he reveals his interest in the details of their medical, social and political features. To this he adds accounts of epidemic outbreaks of other diseases that usually

---

England and Germany, and to the low frequency of the disease in the Spanish army, in which vaccination was mandatory (81). In the same year (1902) Ángel Pulido was laceratingly critical of this deficiency in Spanish and Madrid's public health (*Sanidad* 78).

66 "epidemias locales [...] nada infrecuentes, por la negligencia tradicional de los ciudadanos" (536).

67 *Prensa* 417.

68 "el suelo de la ciudad debe ser propicio a la difusión de la epidemia colérica, por la excesiva humedad" (*Prensa* 464). It was at this time that Pettenkofer famously swallowed a live culture of cholera bacilli provided by Koch to demonstrate that the bacillus, on its own and without predisposing soil (*telluric*) factors, did not cause the disease. He did, in fact, remain unscathed though the *Vibrio* was later isolated from his stools. It is now surmised that Pettenkofer had previously acquired immunity to the bacillus as a result of an unrecognized, subclinical infection.

69 *Prensa* 465–66.

maintain a lower, endemic, profile. He is aware of the miasmatic, telluric and bacterial explanations for epidemics, and reveals a most judicious restraint in his account of the uproar that surrounded Ferrán. He recognizes the prevailing ignorance of the pathological processes underlying diseases, reflecting the uncertainty of informed medical circles. He is also able to identify areas where further evidence is needed before a definitive opinion can be reached. Such measured and informed reporting of the cholera epidemics reflects his profound interest in their medical and social contexts.[70]

70 Fernández Sanz refers, in the context of Galdós's masterly account of the cholera epidemic of 1885, that Galdós wrote, "a chronicle, one might say a complete one, of the facts [of the epidemic], especially accurate in its medical detail and overall an account of exceptional perceptiveness," "una crónica, diríase completa, de la cuestión, especialmente precisa en el aspecto médico y toda ella trasunta de excepcional agudeza" (231).

CHAPTER 3

Endemic Diseases: Tuberculosis, Syphilis and Angina

Unlike the epidemic diseases that spring to public attention by the sudden appearance of unusually large numbers of victims, endemic diseases, *endemias*, maintain a lower profile but a relatively constant presence in the community. In Galdós's Madrid there were many endemic diseases, typhoid and typhus among them, in addition to the legion infections that primarily affected children, the subject of Chapter 7. Two great endemic diseases of adults that Galdós portrays in his novels are tuberculosis and syphilis. Neither disease varied with the seasons and both appeared in all levels of society. While endemic diseases did not cause the kind of panic that outbreaks of cholera inspired, the continuous but less dramatic erosion of the population by tuberculosis, for instance, resulted in more deaths over time.[1]

Understanding of the cause of tuberculosis evolved during the course of Galdós's writing career, notably following Robert Koch's announcement of his discovery of the responsible organism, *Mycobacterium tuberculosis*, in 1882. The disease had been observed to run in families for centuries and was perceived to have increased by the 1880s such that it accounted for 20% of the overall mortality of the population.[2] It was recognized as being associated with the crowding seen in the poorly ventilated hovels of the urban poor, and among soldiers housed in military barracks. In addition, it was thought to be the result of familial predisposition or diathesis, which, in turn, was considered to be a feature of inherited degeneration.[3] So

1 Lloréns y Gallard (9) records in 1900 that deaths from tuberculosis in Barcelona during the two previous decades totalled 22,000, in comparison with the deaths from cholera in the four epidemics in the city that totalled "only" 14,000.

2 Hauser, *siglo* 218.

3 Hauser, *siglo* 220.

rooted was this idea that some, like Hauser in 1885, regarded tuberculosis as having a purifying role for the human race by ridding it of biologically inferior stock.[4]

By 1902, Hauser had incorporated Koch's discovery into his epidemiological account though continues to emphasize environmental factors such as poverty and the foul smells, *mefitismo urbano*, which he claims were much more pronounced in Madrid than in other European capitals.[5] As with almost all other infections, the death rates from tuberculosis were highest in the squalid *barrios* of *Hospicio*, *Latina*, *Inclusa*, *Palacio* and *Universidad*. Hauser suggests that the extremes of the Madrid climate in conjunction with *madrileños*' fondness for night-life in poorly ventilated, crowded places contributed to this mortality.[6]

Galdós's remarkably detailed depiction of pulmonary tuberculosis occurs in the second part of *El doctor Centeno*. In this half of the novel, Felipe Centeno leaves behind the school and family of Pedro Polo as he serves a new master, the genial but recklessly improvident student, Alejandro Miquis. Felipe faithfully follows his master in his descent from the boarding house of doña Virginia to a series of much poorer lodgings. Alejandro's poor constitution is emphasized early on, "physically he was weak with a poor constitution and the fatal habit of squandering his feeble physical resources. He was always highly strung."[7] Galdós's picture is of a degenerate physique associated with an abnormal temperament, both implicitly predisposing his character to disease. It is not long before his obsession with writing an epic drama exhausts him and he starts to lose

4 *siglo* 218. Gutiérrez Jiménez in 1875 also speculates that tuberculosis might serve the purpose of weeding out the weak, *un medio de eliminación de las razas degeneradas*. (181) Darwin expressed similar musings in relation to smallpox (*Descent* 138) well before his cousin, Francis Galton, coined the word *eugenic* in 1883.

5 *Madrid* 128–30.

6 *Madrid* 131.

7 "Fisicamente era raquítico y de constitución muy pobre, con la fatalidad de ser dado a derrochar sus escasas fuerzas vitales. Sus nervios siempre estaban en grado muy alto de tensión" (Pérez Galdós, *Centeno* 321). Citations of *El doctor Centeno* are from the text edited by Román Román, hereafter referred to as *Centeno*.

weight dramatically, "… ending up with an unhealthy loss of weight. He would lie down shattered with fatigue, and was somewhat affected with delirium and with painful attacks of shivering."[8] Alejandro loses his appetite, continues to lose weight and, ominously, is kept awake at night by a painful cough (334). Unable to afford the current rented room, he moves to a squalid garret, but still prowls the night streets only to return one evening, "coughing with such force that he looks as if he is going to tear apart his chest […] his breathing is a harsh whistle, his brow wet with sweat."[9] He suffers a high fever and is delirious and his end is clearly not far off, for he relieves a sense of obstruction in his chest by coughing up a large quantity of blood (375). He moves to even cheaper and worse lodgings, a garret that is managed by the sister of *La Tal*, his prostitute-girl friend. Alejandro is finally seen by the sympathetic doctor, Moreno Rubio (428), who describes to Cienfuegos, the medical student who accompanies him, the features of the breath sounds that he hears on auscultation of the chest. Galdós, as narrator, sings praises of the sounds that can be heard through a stethoscope:

> The sibilant and deep sounds, the echoes, the blows, the quivering and resonant [sounds], diminished and indistinct, that do not resemble a corporeal voice so much as the soliloquies of the soul […]! It is such a pity that the burden of this music is almost always a lament of death! To the [ears of the] listening doctor are conveyed the sighs of the dying.[10]

Galdós does not stop at this evocation, but proceeds to reveal, through Moreno Rubio's conversation with Cienfuegos, his own knowledge of

8 "concluía en enfermizo marasmo. Se acostaba rendido de fatiga, y le entraba algo de delirio, con escalofríos muy penosos" (*Centeno* 327).

9 "rompió a toser con tanta fuerza, que parecía que se le desgarraba el pecho […] Su resuello era un áspero silbido, su frente estaba empapada en tibio sudor" (*Centeno* 374).

10 "La resonancia sibilante, la cavernosa, los ecos, los golpes, los trémulos, las sonoridades, indistintas y apianadas, que ya no parecen voces del cuerpo sino soliloquios del alma ¡Lástima que la letra de esta música sea casi siempre una endecha de muerte! Los oídos del médico se regalan con los suspiros del moribundo" (*Centeno* 428). This lyrical and enthusiastic evocation of breath sounds heard with a stethoscope strongly suggests that Galdós had been given an opportunity to hear them for himself.

the clinical signs and pathological processes associated with advanced pulmonary tuberculosis:

> poor kid! The tubercles have destroyed almost all the [lung] parenchyma. The liquefaction and expulsion of tuberculous material has begun alarmingly. [...] The bronchophonia indicates the sudden formation of large cavities ... We will listen tomorrow and you will be able to observe the curious phenomenon of pectoriloquy ...[11]

The terms bronchophonia (Greek: *bronchus*=windpipe, *phone*=sound) and pectoriloquy (Latin: *pectus*=chest, *loqui*=to speak) are coinages of René Laennec (1781–1826), the father of chest medicine. He used the terms to describe sounds heard through his invention, the stethoscope, which he had devised in 1818. In bronchophonia, the sound of air passing through the air passages is unusually well heard because lung next to the chest wall is abnormally solid (consolidated), with the result that it conducts sound better than does normal air-containing lung. A common cause of this finding in Laennec's (and Galdós's) day was lobar pneumonia, although any pneumonia, such as that resulting from tuberculosis, could produce the same effect. In pectoriloquy, on the other hand, Laennec observed not the breath sounds but the sound of a patient's voice, which was abnormally well-transmitted to the chest wall as a result of a lung cavity immediately underlying the chest wall. A similar speech sound can be heard when the stethoscope is placed on the neck overlying the patient's larynx and vocal cords.[12]

11 "¡pobre chico! Los tubérculos han destruido casi todo el parénquima. Ha empezado de una manera alarmante el reblandecimiento y expulsión de tubérculos. [...] –La broncofonía nos indica la formación súbita de grandes cavernas ... Mañana auscultaremos, y observará usted el curioso fenómeno de la pectoriloquia ..." (*Centeno* 428–29).

12 It follows from the above explanation that Galdós confuses the two entities since it is pectoriloquy that indicates the presence of a cavity, not bronchophonia. This distinction is clearly made by Barrier in 1843 (180) and Latham in 1836 (426–29). With time, the distinction between Laennec's neologisms has become blurred, however, so that at least one modern medical dictionary lists them as synonyms. Galdós's intention in this passage is, of course, that his readers should be impressed by Moreno Rubio's technical, clinical acumen.

At a time when the only confirmation of anatomical lung disease had been that at autopsy, the analysis of breath and voice sounds was a great advance, since it made possible a new precision in following the progress of lung disease in the living patient. Pneumonia and tuberculosis were foremost among the pathological processes that could be assessed by the new technique. In the nineteenth century, clinicians recognized that the formation of lung cavities in tuberculosis, with its resulting pectoriloquy, was of grave import, one of them stating "Where it [the lung cavity] clearly and unequivocally exists, it is unquestionably pathognomonic [...] may announce the speedy approach of suffering, and sorrow, and death ..."[13] It is clear that Moreno's recognition of pectoriloquy in the unfortunate Alejandro correctly identifies him as being mortally ill.

The painful decline of the starving Alejandro continues as, breathless and ever weaker, he lapses into coma and hallucinates, seeing vivid scenes from his epic drama, *El Grande Osuna*. The heat in his garret becomes insufferable (455) and Alejandro is wracked by violent coughing (470) finally feeling no pain as he drowsily lapses into final unconsciousness and death (495), leaving Felipe to lament "he lost his health and his life. Cursed tuberculosis!" (497).

Robert Koch's identification of *Mycobacterium tuberculosis* in 1882 accounted not only for tuberculosis of the lungs but also for the condition of enlarged, ulcerating lymph nodes of the neck, scrofula. The latter disease had been recognized for centuries and was commonplace in the cities of Western Europe, but it was only after Koch's discovery that it was realized that the underlying cause was identical to that of pulmonary tuberculosis. However, the significance of Koch's discovery was assimilated slowly in Spain, as in the rest of Europe, since it had long been believed that pulmonary tuberculosis (*phthisis*) was the result of hereditary, degenerative predisposition. Such a belief is expressed by the physician, Augusto Miquis (Alejandro's brother), in a later novel by Galdós, "an illness of the family,

13 John Forbes *et al.* 233–34. *Pathognomonic:* a sign or symptom, or (later) a laboratory finding, by which a disease may be diagnosed; specifically characteristic or indicative of a particular disease or disorder (Oxford English Dictionary (OED)).

which is perpetuated and transmitted in it [...] like inherited tuberculosis."[14] The real-life physician, the degenerationist *alienista* Escuder, perceived a link between inherited mental instability and inter-generational tuberculosis, "these people with nervous diseases clearly inherit tuberculosis [...] condemning their children to the classic form of pulmonary tuberculosis."[15] This perspective seems particularly applicable to Alejandro with his overwrought imagination and poor grasp of everyday practical matters, a condition in the borderland between eccentricity and insanity that he shares with his great aunt Isabel Godoy.

Galdós must have seen contemporaries with tuberculosis, and a review of contemporary writings on the disease confirms the fidelity of his description. The social and medical features of his description of Alejandro include almost all the factors thought to predispose to the disease in the 1880s. Galdós is unsparing in his description of the utter squalor to which Alejandro and Felipe are reduced. He emphasizes Alejandro's poor physique, the limited resources of energy at his command, and the recklessness with which he squanders them (321). Just such features are described by Moreno Fernández in 1889, who characterizes the predisposed, tubercular type as, "the exaggeration of the lymphatic-nervous temperament[16] seen in infancy and early youth, and above all if combined

14 "un mal de familia, que se perpetuaba y transmitía en ella como [...] la tisis hereditaria" (Pérez Galdós, *Lo prohibido*, Cátedra edition, edited by James Whiston, 136, hereafter cited as *prohibido*).

15 "Estos neurópatas, hereden manifiestamente la tuberculosis [...] engarzando á sus hijos en la forma clásica de la tuberculosis pulmonar" (*Plus* 296). Belief in this association persisted amongst doctors for at least 50 years after Koch's discovery of the *Mycobacterium*, illustrated by the appearance of an article in *The Lancet*, "The Atavistic-Degenerative Diathesis of Tuberculosis" by Rivers in 1923.

16 The 1884 edition of the *Diccionario de la Real Academia Española* defines temperamento as "Predominance of one or other of the three systems nervous, sanguine or lymphatic," "Predominio de uno u otro de los tres sistemas nervioso, sanguíneo o linfático". The theory of temperaments (or humours) goes back to classical times and was summarized by Pedro Monlau in his *Elementos de higiene privada* in 1864, "they consist of disproportions or disequilibria: they are fundamentally true morbid predispositions," "consisten en desproporciones ó en desequilibrios: son en el fondo

with abnormal or perverse sexual activity."[17] Explaining the prostration attributable to excessive sexual activity, he continues, "the sperm cell is an element equal or similar to the nerve [cell]: loss of semen leads to loss of energy and loss of life [...] a hallmark of psychological debility, which is the very essence of predisposition to tuberculosis."[18] A similar view is expressed by Gutiérrez Jiménez in 1875, when he attributes deterioration of the lungs and nervous system to sexual excess, especially that related to prostitution (187).

In recommending measures to prevent tuberculous infection, Gutiérrez lists the very opposite of all the elements that Galdós describes in Alejandro's surroundings: space, cleanliness, healthy food, good ventilation with clean air, avoidance of mental and emotional overstimulation, and harmonious equilibrium of bodily function and intellectual energy (197–204). Gutiérrez specifically counsels avoidance of mental overstimulation, "Beware reading literature that deals greatly with the emotions for it awakes feelings that would be better left unaroused."[19] In *El doctor Centeno*, Galdós clearly links

verdaderas predisposiciones morbosas" (497). His description of the *nervioso* is especially pertinent to Alejandro, "an exquisitely sensitive and impressionable physiology [...] slender and easily fatigued [...] much disposed to art and literature [...] corresponding with an erotic or genital temperament, which at times leads to the pathological," "una exquisita sensibilidad de toda la economía y una grande impresionabilidad, [...] delgado de cuerpo; sus músculos están muy poco pronunciados; el menor ejercicio le fatiga [...] mucha disposición para las bellas artes y la literatura [...] resulta el temperamento erótico ó genital, que llega á veces hasta la morbosidad" (498–90). Routh in 1876 recommends assessment using the criteria of temperaments in the selection of wet-nurses (264–66).

17 "la exageración del temperamento linfático-nervioso, propio de la infancia y del principio de la juventud, sobre todo, si a él se llega por el uso inmoderado, anormal o vicioso de la función generadora" (59). The word "cholera" in the sense of temperament derives from the belief in an excess of yellow bile (Greek: *kholē*=bile).

18 "la célula espermática es un elemento igual o semejante al nervioso: perdiendo semen, se pierden fuerzas, se pierden vida [...] un sello de empobrecimiento anímico, que es la forma más viva y perfecta de la predisposición tuberculosa" (63).

19 "Mucho cuidado con la lectura de obras que, hablando mucho a los sentidos, exciten demasiado su sensibilidad, que conviene mantener dormido" (203).

Alejandro's sexual excesses with his failing energies, tuberculosis and death, suggesting that he was well aware of contemporary medical opinion. One might even be forgiven for imagining that he might have consulted a text such as that of Gutiérrez Jiménez before portraying so many of the risk factors then thought to predispose to tuberculous disease.

Other references to disease in *El doctor Centeno* add resonance to the story of Alejandro's decline. As a diverting counterpoint, Galdós has Felipe repeating what he has must have heard about Alejandro, in relation to a neighbour Rosita's dying cat. Apparently without understanding the significance of the phrase, he diagnoses the moribund young cat as suffering from, "the abuses of youth" (435). On dissecting the animal after its death, he pays particular attention to the lungs, imagining that the cat has died of Alejandro's disease, and repeatedly uses a term for lung tissue, *parénquima*, a word that Moreno Rubio has just used to explain the tuberculous process to Cienfuegos (428). The parallel continues as he finds the cat's stomach empty, "you have not eaten in many days" (437).

The echoes of Alejandro's fatal predicament do not stop here since Galdós inserts a passage describing other manifestations of hunger and poverty in the four children of his neighbour, José Ido de Sagrario, who live in the same building. He gives one a limp, another bowed legs suggestive of rickets, the third a hare-lip and the oldest round shoulders. All are pale, undernourished and suffer from various manifestations of scrofula. They are a cue for Galdós's anguished lament for the "great sickness of our race" (431) that is all the more inexcusable for its being preventable by the measures of good hygiene, fresh air and decent housing. The need for these was well understood at the time, but remained unimplemented.

Seven years after the publication of *El doctor Centeno*, Galdós devotes much of one of his articles for *La Prensa* of Buenos Aires to recent developments in the understanding and treatment of tuberculosis. He reports the introduction by Koch of a novel "lymph" for the treatment of the disease. This appeared to control tuberculous osteomyelitis and the milder forms of chest disease, though was apparently without effect upon advanced pulmonary disease. While describing the great interest of physicians and patients, who are migrating to Berlin in large numbers to study or to receive the serum, Galdós cautions against "premature enthusiasm." He sagely adds that, "problems of this nature require repeated confirmation before they can be regarded as satisfactorily resolved."[20]

Galdós goes on to credit Koch with cures for diphtheria and tetanus citing his research assistants, Behring and "Kilasabo,"[21] as having infected rats with the former disease. He humorously comments on the extraordinary therapeutic powers of rat blood in preventing diphtheria in the porcupine (*Prensa* 441), and cites a wag who suggests that humans injected with rat serum ran the risk of being eaten by cats (442). Galdós's interest in medical detail continues, as he describes the contrasting method of preparing a serum against tetanus that involves the use of rabbits.

In addition to his reportage of medical detail, Galdós meditates on more general medical themes that have a strikingly modern ring to them. He speculates that quantities of benign invading microbes might be ingested to devour pathological ones, "the touchstone of modern therapy is to enable the good against the bad, or to ingest armies of bacilli that consume those [organisms] that harm us."[22] Equally thoughtful is his suggestion that the apparent proliferation of diseases seen by his contemporaries may not be due to diminished resistance of a declining race so much as the result of the improved communication and better statistics, such that the true state of affairs is more evident than previously (*Prensa* 436), a perennial truth no less relevant today.

In common with all major European cities a second endemic disease that had an increasing presence in Galdós's Madrid was syphilis. Like tuberculosis, it afflicted all classes within society, though it was associated in the

20 "problemas de esta naturaleza requieren pruebas muy repetidas para darse por satisfactoriamente resueltos" (*Prensa* 437). Alas, Galdós's caution was fully justified by events since, within a month, Virchow published findings showing that the Koch's lymph (tuberculin) was ineffective in killing the *Mycobacterium*.

21 The correct version of the Japanese bacteriologist's name appears to be Kitasato (Shibasaburō).

22 "el toque de la terapéutica moderna está en dar armas a los buenos contra los malos, o en ingerirnos ejércitos de bacillus que devoran a los que nos causan daño" (*Prensa* 437). A prophetic observation since more recently mixtures of "good" gut flora have sometimes been given to displace disease-producing organisms in the intestine.

popular mind with the impoverished lower classes, especially in relation to prostitution. As with the pulmonary and scrofulous forms of tuberculosis, the common cause of some manifestations of syphilitic disease was not widely appreciated. This was especially so in the delayed (tertiary) disease affecting the nervous system. As had been the case in tuberculosis, the diagnosis was purely clinical, as there were no laboratory tests that could resolve a clinical suspicion. Inevitably, this led to many instances in which the diagnosis could only be confirmed after the disease had progressed, or at autopsy. In both syphilis and tuberculosis hereditary transmission was assumed. In the context of congenital syphilis, there was a widespread (and incorrect) belief that the unborn child could be infected by the father without infection being present in the mother. Unlike tuberculosis, the responsible organism in syphilis was not known in the 1880s, and recognition of the disease was bedevilled by the potentially long latent period between its secondary and tertiary forms that could last for many years.[23] Such latency after treatment could be misinterpreted as a successful cure, making assessment of the efficacy of medications difficult. Treatment with drugs, often containing mercury and iodide, was often associated with suppression of outward manifestations of the disease without halting its underlying, latent progression.

The problems related to venereal disease were compounded by the fact that reference to it was taboo in polite society such that it was often mentioned obliquely, if at all. Open discussion of sexual matters in general

23 The division of syphilitic symptoms and signs into three stages was devised by the French venereologist Philippe Ricord (Crissey and Parish 87). As a gross simplification, primary syphilis takes the form of an ulcer (chancre), secondary a variety of skin rashes, while the tertiary form can involve any part of the body in a bewildering variety of manifestations of which diseases of the central nervous system and aorta are typical. More recently an additional "latent" (asymptomatic) stage between the second and the third stages has been accepted, though the phenomenon of latency in syphilis was described in 1860 by Yvaren, who listed the variety of diseases that syphilis was thought to mimic (499). *Tabes dorsalis* was long considered to be distinct from syphilis. The connection began to be suspected when Fournier published his clinical findings in 1876, but was not be confirmed bacteriologically until the twentieth century.

was considered offensive, and Galdós's own reticence on the topic is well illustrated by his critique of *La Regenta* written to Alas in 1885. Galdós writes, "as this [the act of reproduction] is only seen on certain and limited occasions [...] the book, in my opinion, should provide a similar veil."[24] The penalties for infringement of this taboo could be severe, as one of the more radical Naturalist writers of the time, Eduardo López Bago, discovered when he found himself prosecuted for public indecency after writing about brothel life in *La prostituta* in 1884.[25] José Ortega Munilla, author, journalist and close friend of Galdós, reflected accepted values of his time when he wrote of *La prostituta*, "If it were permissible to discuss prohibited matters we would sample señor López Bago" and accuses the author of an "obscene" Naturalism that paints, "humanity mired in vice and surrounded by brothels, hospitals and markets of sex as if man [...] were not able to apply a major endowment of virtue to oppose this accumulation of evils."[26]

Even in medical texts designed to educate the public, the taboo word *syphilis* might be avoided as being unacceptably offensive. This is illustrated by Tolosa Latour when he edited his doctoral thesis on child and infant care for the guidance of mothers-to-be. In *El Niño*, he warns mothers of the vital importance of sound health in both parents in producing healthy children (29–30), and the danger to infants of contracting syphilis by suckling infected wet-nurses (73). At no point in its 200 pages, however, does Tolosa identify the infection by name, referring to it as a "certain terrible disease [...] the name of which we do not wish to pronounce" (90). A more obscure circumlocution occurs later when he refers to, "that terrible contagious illness described by Fracastor (that we do not wish to name by

24 "como este [el acto de la reproducción] no aparece sino en ciertas y determinadas ocasiones [...] el libro debe, a mi juicio, ofrecer una veladura semejante" (*Alas* 229–30).

25 Pura Fernández 37.

26 "Si fuera lícito discutir sobre cosas prohibidas se lo probaríamos al señor López Bago. [...] una humanidad encenagada en vicios y rodeada de lupanares, hospitales y lonjas de amor, como si los hombres [...] contra esta cuenta de maldades no pudiesen oponer una considerable data de virtudes" (2).

its *nom de guerre* when discussing marriage and [...] next to a crib where all should be purity)."[27]

Other medical writers, however, were prepared to be more frank in their writing for the general public, and Hauser was one of them. In his 1885 review of public health in Spain in the *Revista de España*, he cites the disease by name and continues, "Its devastating increase in the last 50 years is truly frightening, involving every social group, both sexes and all ages, either by direct contact or by heredity; one can consequently call it a social disease specific to our century being one of the factors weakening and degenerating the human race."[28] He emphasizes the well-recognized link between syphilis and prostitution with the translation of a passage written by the great French hygienist, Parent-Duchatelet, "Of all the contagious diseases harmful to society that can affect the human race, there is none more serious, more dangerous or more fearsome than syphilis".[29] It should be added that the extent of the disease in society was worse than

27 "aquella terrible y contagiosa enfermedad cantada por Fracastor (que no quisimos llamar por su *nombre de guerra* cuando hablábamos del matrimonio, y [...] junto à una cuna, donde debe ser todo pureza)" (62, my italics). Girolamo Fracastoro (about 1477–1553) was an Italian physician and poet famous in medical history for his epic poem of 1530 about a shepherd named *Syphilus* who insulted Apollo and was punished with a horrible disease (Quétel 52–53). Frascatoro lived through the period when syphilis appeared in Naples after Columbus's return from the New World, and subsequently spread throughout Europe with the initial speed of an epidemic, a characteristic of infections in populations previously unexposed to them (Crosby 219). One wonder how many of Tolosa's readers would have understood his erudite reference to the Italian. In contrast, when he was addressing an audience made up entirely of medical men, Tolosa felt quite able to name the otherwise unmentionable disease (*Protección* 19–20).

28 "Es verdaderamente asombroso su incremento desolador en los últimos cincuenta años, invadiendo todas las capas sociales, todas las edades y sexos, ya por transmisión, ya por herencia; y por lo tanto, puede llamarse una enfermedad social propia de nuestro siglo, constituyendo uno de los agentes debilitantes y degenerativos de la raza humana" (*siglo* 214).

29 "De todas las enfermedades que pueden afectar á la especie humana por vía de contagio y que traen perjuicios á la sociedad, no hay ninguna más grave, más peligrosa ni más temible que la sífilis" (215).

Hauser and his contemporaries realized since it was not known that the common spinal affliction of *tabes dorsalis* and the cerebral disease of G.P.I. were both syphilitic in origin, though a link was suspected by Fournier.[30] Hauser was not alone in his fears as his contemporary, Enrique Gelabert, made the astonishing assertion that, "syphilis on its own causes more devastation than all other infectious diseases together,"[31] while the Barcelona venereologist, José Viñeta-Bellaserra, echoed Hauser's fear that syphilis was the cause of national, biological degeneration (*punible* 49).

This environment of fear and censorship presented Galdós with a problem. His announced ambition in 1870 had been to portray all aspects of the middle class, which he saw as the driving force in Spanish society.[32] However, he could not risk alienating his readers, or worse still, provoke the authorities into banning publication of his work, as happened to López Bago. He solved this dilemma with finesse by sowing the texts of his novels with indirect references that would be understood by those of his readers with experience of the world, without offending others who might be upset by details that they found too graphic. This distinction could be a difficult one to draw. While in some of his descriptions characters' telltale oddities are subtle and easily missed, his great portrait of congenital syphilis in Maximiliano Rubín in *Fortunata y Jacinta* is graphic and almost repellent in its veracity.[33]

The profile of Maximiliano begins with family history and details of his late mother. She was beautiful, lived beyond her husband's means, led a scandalous life and had three sons who looked so completely different

30 In the same article, Hauser claims that 20–25% of patients in asylums in all European countries suffered from G.P.I. (206). At the beginning of the twentieth century, according to Herrera Hernández, syphilis was estimated to affect about 15% of the European population, while *tabes dorsalis* was one of the most important and common neurological diseases then seen (*Perspectivas* 507).

31 "la sífilis causaba por sí sola más estragos que todas las enfermedades contagiosa juntas" (25).

32 *Observaciones* 167.

33 The substance of the passages that follow is dealt with in more detail in Stannard (*Rubín*).

from each other to suggest that they had different fathers (*I* 448–49).[34] The implication of sexual promiscuity is clear. All brothers have severe headaches. Maxi was weakly and unattractive as a child, has a lymphatic constitution, and was born at seven months' gestation, when he needed to be fed with a bottle and by a goat (*I* 459–50).[35] As an adult, he has a poor memory with the result that his attempts at study are arduous. He has such a feeble body that it seems as if the wind might blow him over, and has a flattened head, lank hair and premature balding. Very strikingly, the bridge of his nose has collapsed, his teeth are very irregular, he suffers from bone pain and he has severe catarrh.[36] Maxi medicates himself with

34 The citations of *Fortunata y Jacinta* are from the two-volume *Cátedra* edition edited by Francisco Caudet hereafter cited as *Fortunata I* and *II*.

35 "Maximiliano era raquítico, de naturaleza pobre y linfática, absolutamente privado de gracias personales. Como que había nacido de siete meses y luego se le criaron con biberón y con una cabra" (*Fortunata I* 459–60). Monlau lists the features of the lymphatic temperament: "soft swollen flesh, fine colourless, hairless skin, lank hair, slow pulse, easily depressed, slow and laborious in movement, sleeping long and deeply," "carnes blandas y abotagadas; piel fina, descoloradas, sin velo [...] cabellos lisos [...] pulso lento, blando, fácil de deprimir [...] movimientos tardíos, lentos y penosos; sueño largo y profundo" (*Elementos* 542). Galdós writes specifically "se le criaron [...] con una cabra," signifying not that he was merely fed with goat's milk (as has appeared in a translation of the novel) but that he was actually suckled by a goat.

36 "the bony [bridge] of his nose was sunken and flattened as if it were of soft material and had received a blow, resulting not only in ugliness but also in obstruction of nasal breathing, which was without doubt the cause of his mouth always being open. His teeth had erupted so unequally that each tooth was, as one might say, where it pleased. And if only those damned bones did not ever trouble him. The poor thing had such toothache that he could cry to the heavens. He also suffered infections of the nose that followed one after another resulting in a chronic rhinitis," "Tenía el hueso de la nariz hundido y chafado, como si fuera de sustancia blanda y hubiese recibido un golpe, resultando de esto no sólo fealdad sino obstrucciones de respiración nasal, que eran sin duda la causa de que tuviera siempre la boca abierta. Su dentadura había salido con tanta desigualdad que cada pieza estaba, como si dijéramos, donde le daba la gana. Y menos mal si aquellos condenados huesos no le molestaran nunca; ¡pero si tenía el pobrecito cada dolor de muelas que le hacía poner el grito más allá

every known form of potassium iodide.[37] In addition he appears to suffer from delayed sexual development since he looks much younger than his 25 years and has no moustache.[38]

Maxi is mentally unstable and becomes obsessed with the idea that he has an aneurysm of the aorta that ruptures, dreaming that it floods the room with his blood (*I* 220–21). He contemplates murder-suicide (*I* 703), is convinced that his family wants to poison him (*II* 279), has a mania for logical analysis (*II* 417) and suffers from delusions of religious grandeur.[39] He experiences a hallucination of a nocturnal intruder (*II* 277) and tries to murder the cook (*II* 385). In a later lucid interval, he is able objectively to summarize the features of his psychosis (*II* 491).[40]

The reactions of those about Maxi are also revealing. Both his older brother, Juan, and Maxi's pharmaceutical mentor, Ballester, speculate that he may benefit from medication known to help those with diffuse peri-encephalitis or meningoencephilitis (*II* 399), while Maxi's aunt, doña Lupe, confides to her daughter-in-law, Fortunata, that Ballester has revealed to her that he thinks Maxi may have softening of the brain (*II* 259).

Galdós here presents us with a clinical *tour de force* that reveals knowledge of contemporary medicine. The complex of features he details indicates that he had a specific disease in mind, since it corresponds closely with the

del Cielo! Padecía también de corizas y las empalmaba, de modo que resultaba un coriza crónico" (*Fortunata I* 456).

37 "he dosed himself with every possible form of potassium iodide," "se administraba el ioduro de potasio en todas las formas posibles" (*Fortunata I* 456).

38 "Maximiliano was twenty five years old but did not look more than twenty. He had no moustache," "tenía Maximiliano veinticinco y no representaba más de veinte. Carecía de bigote" (*Fortunata I* 458).

39 "I am no more than the forerunner of this doctrine: its true Messiah will come later; he will come soon, he is already on the way. He who knows everything has told me," "Yo no soy más que el precursor de esta doctrina; el verdadero Mesías de ella vendrá después, vendrá pronto; ya está en camino. Quien todo se lo sabe me lo ha dicho a mí" (*Fortunata II* 307).

40 Psychosis: A severe mental disease characterized by loss of contact with reality (in the form of delusions and hallucinations) and deterioration of intellectual and social functioning (OED).

description of the English physician, Jonathan Hutchinson (1828–1913), who was one of the great experts in venereal disease of his day.[41] In 1858, Hutchinson had published an account of a previously unrecognized form of congenital syphilis, one that presented not in infancy, as that was already well-known, but in adult life.

Infection of mother and child with a history of repeated miscarriages, prematurity, or death of children in infancy had been recognized since the epidemic spread of syphilis from Naples in the 1490s. Infants surviving into childhood often died despite treatment with a variety of medications, which often contained mercury. By the nineteenth century, crowding and poverty in rapidly growing cities, linked with prostitution, were associated with a fearsome increase in venereal disease that physicians were obliged to confront. As Hutchinson did so, he recognized signs and symptoms of advanced (*tertiary*) syphilis in a group of patients in adolescence and early adulthood, which prompted him to ask when the infection had been acquired, whether during infancy from an infected wet-nurse, for instance, or from before birth.

Hutchinson made the key observation that affected patients' permanent teeth were consistently malformed, which indicated that their development had been disrupted during intrauterine life. This proved that this form of tertiary syphilis had to be congenital, with its sufferers unusually surviving to be seen by a doctor in adolescence or adult life. Hutchinson places particular emphasis upon these dental irregularities, one variety of whch has been associated with his name in medicine ever since.[42] In addition, Hutchinson describes short stature, skin that may appear thin and hair that is thin and dry. He lists disease of the bones and joints, while the sunken and flattened nose he describes as "a very marked condition in most cases and constitutes a very valuable sign" (265). He ends by asserting

41 I once presented this literary portrait as an "unknown" at a clinical case conference to a group of infectious disease specialists. They had no difficulty in making the diagnosis.

42 Hutchinson's teeth: small, rounded, pegged or screwdriver-shaped incisors that are notched on their cutting edge. An associated, typical, dome-shaped deformity of the first molar teeth was described by Henry Moon (1845–92).

the prime importance of the *tout ensemble*, such that, "it is not by any one symptom that the diagnosis of hereditary syphilis can ever be supported but by the careful estimation of the entire group" (265). His observations were confirmed by the France venereologist, Alfred Fournier (1832–1914), who published his findings in 1886.[43] Fournier's clinical experience led him to be so suspicious of young men with severe, chronic headaches that he recommended that chronic, syphilitic meningitis should be considered as a likely cause and be so treated, especially when there was a family history suspicious of the disease (*héréditaire* 488).

Among the other features of delayed congenital syphilis that Galdós gives Maxi are chronic catarrh (coryza), bone pain and prematurity. These were well-known at the time and are described in texts such as that of Georges Homolle (1845–83) (867, 880). A striking feature of Galdós's description is Maxi's obsessive self-treatment with potassium iodide, "in every possible form," since the only indication for this medication listed in the *Farmacopea Oficial Española* of 1884 is, "for particular use in the treatment of the manifestations of tertiary syphilis."[44] A more general use of potassium iodide in the treatment of syphilis is also listed in volume II of the Spanish translation of Christie's *Burroughs Wellcome Blue Book, Libro médico azul*, a copy of which was in Galdós's own library (De la Nuez Caballero 98). The reference to this very specific medication strongly suggests that Galdós is not only hinting to his more knowledgeable readers that Maxi has a particular form of syphilis, but also that Maxi is aware of his condition and that he is doing all he can to treat it. The use of potassium iodide in the treatment of syphilitic patients became more common after 1835 when the Dublin dermatologist-venereologist, William Wallace, recommended it in the treatment of syphilis that did not respond to traditional medications containing compounds of mercury (11). Though this therapeutic innovation had been introduced earlier by Antonio Breva

43 (*héréditaire* 86–94). It should be emphasized that clinicians had no laboratory tests to confirm their findings and had to work entirely on the basis of clinical history and examination. The organism responsible for syphilis, *Treponema pallidum*, was not described until 1905, and a diagnostic test for it not developed until 1906.

44 "de uso especial en el tratamiento de los fenómenos terciarios de la sífilis" (414).

(Crissey and Parish 363), it seems only to have been more widely adopted only after Wallace's publication, with its use extending to Spain following texts such as that of Payan, translated from the French in 1847.

Confirming the suspicion of Maxi's awareness of his condition, Galdós describes him as hypochondriacally obsessed with a complication of tertiary syphilis, an abnormal swelling of the aorta (aneurysm) and its not uncommon complication, rupture, which was always fatal. The association of aneurysmal dilatation of the thoracic aorta with tertiary syphilis was fully documented for the first time in 1875 by the British Army pathologist, Francis Welch, on the basis of autopsies he performed on soldiers who had died in the prime of life.[45] Writing only eleven years after the publication of this paper, Galdós indicates that Maxi knows of this serious complication of his debilitating disease and of its potential for a fatal outcome. From the story of the novel, we may surmise that Maxi has read about thoracic aortic aneurysm in one of the "great medical tomes," *librotes de Medicina*, in the Samaniego/Ballester pharmacy that Fortunata criticises him for reading (*II* 220).

In Maxi's hypochondriacal obsession and intermittently tenuous grasp of reality, Galdós is providing a further clue in view of the suspected a link between syphilis and G.P.I., *parálisis general de los alienados*.[46] The terrible combination of progressive paralysis and dementia was recognized in asylums throughout the Western world following its description by Bayle in 1822 (Ackerknecht, *short* 51; Quétel 160).[47] Word must have reached Spain

45 Welch describes aneurysms of the ascending (first) part of the aorta in the chest. Maxi's imaginary symptoms involve the arm and chest and are consistent with this form of the disease, as is his youth. Aneurysms that involve the aorta in the abdomen usually occur later in life and are the result of different causes. An earlier description of syphilitic aortic aneurysm by Giovanni Lancisi appears to have been forgotten at this time (Crissey and Parish 220).

46 Fournier was not certain at this time that all G.P.I. was due to syphilis and postulated an analogous "pseudo-G.P.I." that was truly syphilitic (*cerveau* xiii leçon). This apparent distinction dissolved in time as he accumulated further case statistics (Quétel 163).

47 In his poll of Spanish *alienistas* in 1882–83, Seguin records that a consensus had observed a striking increase in G.P.I. in the previous 15 years (411).

since a causal relationship between syphilis and *parálisis general* is described by specialists such as Seguin (390, 412) and Vera (33, 37), the latter the colleague of Tolosa Latour. While G.P.I. more commonly occurs in later adult life, sometimes after a latent period of many years, it can also afflict those with the delayed, congenital form of the disease. An account of Galdós's description of Maxi's psychosis attributable to G.P.I. follows in Chapter 5.

Galdós's daringly detailed portrait of syphilis illustrates the strength of his determination to describe features of the middle class that he knew, no matter how unpalatable. It would be incorrect, however, to imagine that Maximiliano Rubín was his only reference to the disease. Subtle references abound in *Fortunata y Jacinta*, such as that of the friend of Feliciana, in a café of dubious repute, who has just been discharged from the hospital of *San Juan de Dios*, Madrid's notorious institution for the treatment of venereal disease (*II* 41).

Galdós's inclusion of the Samaniego-Ballester pharmacy in *Fortunata y Jacinta* gives him repeated opportunities to hint at the prevalence of syphilis in Fortunata's Madrid by narrating customers' need for anti-syphilitic medications that contain iodine (*II* 281), mercury (*II* 319) or a combination of both (*II* 285, 319). In his review of the drugs that appear in part 4 of the novel, Franz lists medications that imply other conditions that were taboo in non-medical literature of the time:

> but this apparent impediment [playing jokes on other characters] to reading the drugs as a guide to Maxi's illnesses disappears once we accept the axiom that the total listing of drugs in Maxi's laboratory contains a code erected to suggest Maxi's secret ailments, including matters that Galdós judged better left to the reader's private detection: impotency, drug dependence, venereal disease, and the like.[48]

In addition, behind the jocular direction that Ballester gives Maxi in the preparation of prescriptions lays an indirect reference to the prostitution that was then regarded as the prime source of syphilitic infection:

> Let us then, dearest colleague, prepare these pills of mercury protoiodide [...] take great care with this precious mercurial. The patient for whom it is prescribed must

48 Franz 43–44.

> be in a real mess. [...] But to tell the truth he must have had a very good time with beautiful women in this world, and if he is paying for it now, he must have had some great times. ¡Hay! ... be careful with the dose. Don't get carried away. You will irritate the patient, and his saliva will flood all over us ...[49]

Galdós's interest in medicine led him to give some of his characters more subtle symptoms associated with venereal disease. In *Lo prohibido* the central character José María describes his cousin, Raimundo, who was once brilliant and charming but has since decayed to a point of exhibiting, "odd enthusiasms and to be regrettably careless about his social and private behaviour."[50] Something has clearly gone fundamentally wrong with him, since though once brilliantly talented he has lost all drive, has been unable to persevere with any career, and is prematurely aged, looking ten years older than his actual 30 years, appearing to anticipate old age (168–69).

In the understanding of the time, he mirrors José María in that he has prematurely exhausted his supplies of energy, "I realized that there was already little oil left in that lamp that had burned early and been stirred up constantly."[51] The implication is that Raimundo has dissipated his energies and is now paying for it. He confirms this in his confession to José María, "I have got the beginning of a serious illness. Do you know what it is? Softening of the spinal cord."[52] He tells José María that there is no need for

49 "Vamos ahora, mi queridísima colega, a hacer estas píldoras de *protoyoduro de mercurio* [...] mucho cuidado con este precioso mercurial. Aviado estará el enfermo para quien sea. [...] Pero a fe que se habrá divertido bastante en este mundo con las mozas guapas, y si buenos azotes le cuesta ahora, buenas ínsulas se habrá calzado. ¡Eh! ... cuidado con la dosis. No sea usted tan vivo de genio. Mire que va a jorobar al paciente, y la saliva que eche va a llegar hasta aquí ..." (*II* 285, author's italics). Excess salivation was a well-known feature of overdose with mercurial drugs. It was characteristic of the age that prostitution was seen as a problem caused by the prostitute rather than the client as Viñeta-Bellaserra, *punible* 52 ff. illustrates.

50 "Tener manías estrambóticas y a padecer lamentables descuidos en su conducta social y privado" (*prohibido* 166).

51 "Comprendí que en aquella lámpara había ya poco aceite, por haber sido encendida muy pronto y atizada constantemente" (*prohibido* 169).

52 "Tengo un principio de enfermedad grave. ¿Sabes lo que es? Reblandecimiento de la médula" (*prohibido* 170)

him to him to consult a doctor as he has already read all about its course, symptoms and treatment (170). After a long discourse with medical terms that José María says he does not understand, Raimundo reveals the symptom that is currently distressing him, that of loss of ability to express himself, "Do you know [...] what is one of the principal symptoms of softening of the spinal cord? Aphasia, that is, loss of the [spoken] word."[53] Like Maxi

53 "¿Sabes [...] cuál es uno de los principales síntomas del reblandecimiento? La afasia, o sea pérdida de la palabra" (*prohibido* 170). Whiston notes the report of a woman with tertiary syphilis and aphasia in Galdós's copy of Armangué y Tuset's *Estudios*, and speculates that Raimundo's aphasia may be a hint that he suffered the same disease (*prohibido* 170 n.56). Armangué dedicated another text, *Mimicismo* (1884), to Giné y Partagas and may have acquired from him the idea of aphasia being due to a tertiary syphilitic mass (gumma) compressing Broca's speech area of the brain. Giné details just such a case in a different patient (*venéreas* 640). In fact, Galdós's hint that Raimundo suffered from syphilis may be a good deal broader than this since, by 1882, *reblandecimiento de la médula* was recognized as being linked with syphilitic *tabes dorsalis*. Fournier describes aphasia in *tabes* where the underlying lesion is diffuse cerebral syphilis in which no focal mass compressing the brain is involved (*l'ataxie* 259, 286, 336).

Despite the disappearance of almost all of Galdós's medical records, there is evidence to suggest that he suffered from *tabes dorsalis* and that this disease contributed to the decline of his later years. The topic has been extensively researched by Herrera Hernández. On the morning of Galdós's death, an unnamed member of Galdós's household revealed to a reporter of *El Figaro* that the author had died of arteriosclerosis and "reblandecimiento medular" (*Muerte de un Gran Español*). Corroboration is provided by Galdós's secretary, friend and fellow Canarian, the journalist Rafael de Mesa, who Ortiz-Armengol describes as, "an unimpeachable biographical authority of those final years," "incuestionable autoridad como biógrafo en estos años finales" (806). In a short biography of Galdós written by de Mesa in 1919 and published on Galdós's death, he writes of the author's blindness, "What caused Galdós's blindness was not the cataracts of his eyes, but the disease called *tabes dorsal*, which in crude Castillian we call softening [of the spinal cord]," "Lo que cegó a D. Benito no fueron los cataratas de sus ojos, sino la enfermedad llamado *tabes dorsal*, que en recio castellano llamamos reblandecimiento" (48, author's italics).

Giné y Partagas, *freno-patología* 533 records dificulty in articulating speech, which he calls *dislalia*, in G.P.I. In Lesson 49 of his text on syphilis, *afasia* appears repeatedly (*venéreas* p. 624 ff.). Vera records having seen similar manifestation of the disease (43).

in *Fortunata y Jacinta*, Raimundo has been reading medical texts and is able to dazzle José María with the technical terms, *terminachos*, acquired as a result of his study, his *lucubración científica* (170). As with Maxi, the technical jargon that Raimundo musters gives us a clue to the kind of condition he has been reading about. The element "cerebral softening," *reblandecimiento*, is particularly significant, as already explained in the context of Maxi Rubín, because by the 1880s, it was becoming apparent that *tabes* was also commonly due to tertiary syphilis. Hammond in 1879 strongly suggests the association (1183), while, by 1882, Fournier was quite convinced of the common, syphilitic cause of the diseases G.P.I. and *tabes dorsalis*.

Galdós thus reveals to his readers with any medical knowledge the likely background of Raimundo's deterioration and his difficulty with speech.[54] His moral and physical decline mirrors that which consumes so many characters in the novel, above all José María himself.

A sense of moral decay is also reflected in the behaviour of Serafín, the retired naval officer and Rafael's brother. Though less information is provided about him than about Raimundo, we learn that he was a hell-raiser in his youth before going to sea. (139) Two features of his life in retirement are striking. Though upright and courteous, in private he is a compulsive kleptomaniac pocketing an extraordinary range of items belonging to others, apparently without being able to control himself. Rafael is at a loss to account for his brother's behaviour, "it's a mystery of nature, a cerebral aberration."[55]

José María confirms this behaviour at his own expense when he finds that possessions such as a book, a small bronze, an ashtray and other knick-knacks are disappearing into the pockets of Serafín's overcoat (175). He

54 Physicians in Galdós's time distinguished *aphasia (dysphasia*, if partial*)* when the patient is unable to conceptualize words, from *dislalia* (*dysarthria*) when the patient knows the words but has difficultly in coordinating the movements of tongue and lips to articulate them. Giné y Partagas describes *dislalia* in G.P.I. (*freno-patología* 537, 543). Examination of Raimundo's speech problem (*prohibido* 170) and the hilarious tongue-twister with which he attempts to cure it (171) suggests that his problem is more one of dysarthria than aphasia.

55 "Es un misterio de la Naturaleza, una aberración cerebral" (*prohibido* 140).

mourns to see such a mean habit develop in a man formerly capable of acts of military valour and reflects, "I believe that he himself did not realize what he was doing, that his light-fingeredness was a neuro-pathological phenomenon, an irresponsible act independent of ideas of the moral."[56] Galdós here hints at a medical background to Serafín's anomalous behaviour, a suggestion that is strengthened by his other hobby, that of compulsive skirt-chasing in the streets, "He who in his mature years had been a high-flying *don Juan*, in old age chased pretty servants, or those who seemed pretty to him, for we must believe that aberrations of taste accompany the affections of senility. His strolls by morning and evening took the form of a feverish, active pursuit that was almost always fruitless."[57] Later in the novel, as he describes his own moral and psychological deterioration, José María, finds that he enjoys the geriatric company of Rafael and Serafín and is amused by Serafín's skirt-chasing and constant ogling of women, which even takes place from their shared box at the bull-ring (573).

Galdós is here vividly describing two forms of behaviour that were associated in his time with G.P.I., a "neuro-pathological phenomenon" if ever there was one. Giné y Partagas describes a patient with the condition as being in, "a continuous erotic fever,"[58] and in reviewing the manifestations of the condition states that patients can, "feel compulsive sexual excitement that leads them to perform obscenities, even in public."[59] Descriptions of *exitación genésica* and *kleptomanía* in G.P.I. appear repeatedly in Vera's monograph on G.P.I., which was published four years before *Lo prohibido* (43, 47, 48, 60, 67). Vera describes in some of the patients he saw, "Sexual

56 "Creo que él mismo no se daba cuenta de lo que hacía; que sus hurtos eran un fenómeno neuropático, un acto irresponsable, independiente de toda idea moral" (*prohibido* 175).

57 "El que en edad madura había sido un galanteador de alto vuelo, en la vejez perseguía a criadas bonitas, o que a él le parecían tales, pues debemos creer que las aberraciones del gusto andarían a la par con la afición senil. Sus paseos matinales y crepusculares eran una cacería activa, febril, casi siempre infructuosa" (*prohibido* 175).

58 "un continuo furor erótico" (*venéreas* 641).

59 "sienten imperiosas excitaciones genitales, que les conducen á cometer obscenidades, aun en público" (*freno-patología* 532).

excitement reaches such intensity and the ability to repeat coitus [becomes] so marked that there are patients of whom one can say that they do nothing other than exercise their sexual functions."[60] Vera mentions patients with kleptomania more than once, "wherever they find themselves, surreptitiously at times, at others indifferent to being observed, they take a wide collection of objects whether they are worth anything or not."[61] Henry Maudsley (1835–1918) in England in 1879 draws a direct connection between kleptomania and G.P.I., emphasizing the subject's lack of criminal responsibility (*Materialism* 247–48). Foville observes that kleptomania is almost always a feature of other conditions, rather than being an isolated condition, and lists G.P.I. as the most common of these (*Kleptomanie* 702).

It seems likely that Galdós was aware of this consensus on erotomania and kleptomania when he crafted his portrait. What is clear is that, even as he depicted comparatively minor characters, Galdós would endow them with pathological features drawn from his extensive knowledge of medicine. In the case of Raimundo and Serafín, such features emphasize the atmosphere of moral and physical decay that pervades *Lo prohibido*.

Among the many other endemic infections prevalent in Galdós's Madrid was that of sore throat. In contrast with the ubiquitous throat infection in the winter months in modern populations, often controlled with antibiotics, the entity labelled as "angina" (Latin: *angina*=quinsy=sore throat) included numerous conditions, some of them chronic and others acute and often fatal.[62] Galdós's edition of Jaccoud lists *angina catarrhal*, which in its chronic form might be associated with scrofula or syphilis, and in the acute version was associated with passing seasonal infection. More serious was the *angina parenquimatosa* that was associated with

60 "La excitación genésica alcanza tanta intensidad y la facilidad para repetir el coito tal grado que hay enfermos de los que puede decirse que no hacen otra cosa que ejercer las funciones genitales" (47).

61 "donde quiera que se halle, con disimulo unas veces, otras sin cuidarse de ser visto, se va apoderando de infinita colección de objetos, valgan ó no valgan" (60).

62 "Angina," derived ultimately from the Greek "strangle," is to be distinguished from the more common present usage of "angina pectoris," which is associated with pain in the chest and the arm, and which is associated with heart disease.

abscess formation behind the pharynx and about the tonsils. The third variety *angina membranosa* described the formation of a false membrane in the larynx and was synonymous with diphtheria, which also bore the name *angina maligna*.[63]

When the beautiful Eloísa in *Lo prohibido* suffers from fever and sore throat, she is given the diagnosis of *angina maligna*. At no time, however, does she suffer from the crowing, croupy respiratory distress that is typical of diphtheria, such as we see in the fatal affliction of Monina in *La familia de León Roch*. Diphtheria was considered to be rare in adults (Hauser, *Madrid II* 87), probably because it was so common in the young, that children either died from it or, or acquired immunity to it on recovery. It is clear that the term *angina maligna* was used to describe more than one variety of severe, sore throat. Details of Galdós's description may help to indicate the condition that he depicts.

He describes Eloísa's customary feeling of a feather in the throat, presumably hysterical, change into something more serious, "Soon a sore throat developed with a very high fever. The doctor said that it was a malignant sore throat. She could not swallow and felt suffocated. Suddenly the neck began to swell … a horrible swelling that increased by the hour, with a rising fever, and consciousness clouded … delirium, restlessness."[64] José María, Eloísa's lover, experiences horror at the sight of her beautiful features so grotesquely deformed:

63 Jaccoud, *II* 628–65. In a footnote, Jaccoud lists *angina maligna* as a synonym of diphtheritic angina (*II* 645). Bouchut and Deprés, in addition to listing angina complicating scarlet fever, also refer to gangrenous, leathery and ulcerating types of anginas as *maligne*, "Angine gangreneuse, angine couenneuse et angine ulcéreuse sont les trois formes anatomiques d'une seule et unique maladie qui est l'angine maligne" (95).

64 "Pronto se determinó una angina, con fiebre intensísima. El médico dijo que era una angina maligna. No podía tragar; se ahogaba. De pronto empezó a hinchársele el cuello … un bulto horrible, que crecía por horas, y la fiebre subiendo, y el cerebro trastornado … delirio, inquietud" (*prohibido 486*). "Maligna" in this context signifies "very serious," rather than cancerous.

> the certainty that the monstrosity was the face that I knew in the fullness of its grace and beauty caused me indescribable terror. It seemed to me an enormous pumpkin in which only the upper part bore any relation to human features. But in the lower part the deformity was such that one would have to resort to the ugliest species of animal to find its like.[65]

Eloísa is very disturbed by her ugliness and persistently high fever, and is not reassured when a relative lies to her about her temperature. We learn that her sister, Camila, has been applying poultices, and that the sound practitioner, Moreno Rubio, predicts recovery with a detailed account of the condition that the narrator, José María, chooses to omit (496). Moreno's prognosis is correct and despite swelling and pain in the face and much emotional distress, Eloísa makes a complete recovery.

Galdós gives a detailed description of severe, painful lower facial and throat swelling with difficulty in swallowing and breathing, but without the croup that is a feature of diphtheria. The clinical picture is not sufficiently detailed to be certain, but a case can be made for Galdós having seen, or been informed about, the condition of Ludwig's angina, one of the conditions referred to at the time, quite justifiably, as *angina maligna*. Wilhelm Ludwig (1790–1865) described the uncommon condition of an inflammatory mass of the floor of the mouth in 1836.[66] Frequently associated with infected teeth, it is a non-abscess forming, inflammatory mass (*phlegmon*) of the tissues below the tongue associated with firm swelling of the neck, high fever and delirium. Swallowing is difficult and there is a sense of suffocation. The crowing respiration of croup may be seen in later stages, but is not typical. The diffuse inflammatory progress may proceed to gangrene and, without modern treatment with antibiotics, is usually fatal. Though Ludwig's angina only appears to be frequent in the French

65 "causome indecible terror la certidumbre de que aquella monstruosidad era la cara que conocí en la plenitud de la gracia y la hermosura. Pareciome enorme calabaza, cuya parte superior era lo único que declaraba parentesco con la fisonomía humana. Mas en la inferior, la deformidad era tal que había que recurrir a las especies zoológicas más feas para encontrarle semejanza" (*prohibido 487*).

66 Ludwig's original description is translated into English, with a biographical note, by John Burke.

medical literature after 1890, it is mentioned in passing in Dechambre's medical dictionary in 1882,[67] and twice in the French translation of Leyden's German text in 1879.[68]

It is difficult to be certain of this identification, partly in view of the variety of conditions to which the term *angina maligna* was applied. As it is not typical of diphtheria, which was very well-known at that time, an acute and serious sore throat with severe swelling of the lower face would be consistent with Ludwig's variety of *angina maligna*. As the condition was fatal almost as often as diphtheria, Eloísa would have been fortunate to survive.

67 "under the name Ludwig's angina, some German authors seem to us to have confused subhyoid phlegmon on the one hand, and sub-maxillary mumps on the other," "sous le nom d'angine de Ludwig, quelques auteurs allemands nous paraissent avoir confondu, d'une part, le phlegmon sus-hyoïdien, d'autre part, les oreillons sous-maxillaires" (*17* 352).

68 "In Mannkopf's patient, the onset [of the condition] was a malignant phlegmonous angina (Ludwig's angina)," "Dans le cas de Mannkopf le début a été une angine phlegmoneuse maligne (angine de Ludwig)" (304). On the following page Leyden discusses the extension of infection into the vertebral canal as a result of various infections and, "more rarely the phlegmonous angina of Ludwig," "plus rarement à l'angine phlegmoneuse de Ludwig" (305). Galdós's friend, the surgeon Alejandro San Martín, was fluent in German as well as in French and English (Goyanes 227). As an admirer of German universities, he would have been in an excellent position to inform Galdós about German medicine.

CHAPTER 4

Alcoholism

It seems likely that Galdós had strong personal feelings about alcohol. Despite being addicted to cigarettes and cigars throughout his adult life, to the extent of defying medical advice and continuing to smoke as he convalesced from cataract surgery, his consumption of alcohol appears to have been negligible.[1] This is all the more remarkable for his being firmly rooted in the social life of the Madrid *tertulias* where much alcohol was consumed as well as coffee.

The social and economic problems of widespread consumption of distilled spirits were inseparable from the growth of cities throughout Europe in the nineteenth century.[2] Wine and beer had been staple items of diet since time immemorial and were often healthier than water supplies as a result of the sterilizing effect of their alcohol content. However, among the industrial advances of the eighteenth and early nineteenth centuries came the development of more efficient and cheaper methods of distillation. These made spirits derived from grain, sugar and root crops much easier and cheaper to produce. In addition the concentration of alcohol

1 "He rebelled against keeping the bandages on and lifted prematurely the doctor's ban on smoking" (Berkowitz, *Pérez* 411). Shoemaker observes, "He followed a regime of eating little and of drinking less, or almost nothing [...] His only great vice was tobacco: he chain-smoked, or sucked and chewed cigars," "Seguía un regimen de comer poco y de beber menos, o casi nada [...] Su único gran vicio era el Tabaco: fumaba, o chupaba y mascaba, puros en cadena" (*Cómo* 6).

2 The medical, social and economic effects of alcoholism in nineteenth-century Spain have been the subject of many recent studies, notably those of Fuentes Peris, and of Campos.

in distilled spirits could be 3–4 times that found in wine, making it much more intoxicating.[3]

Increased consumption of alcohol by the poor and the resulting public drunkenness became a serious problem in cities such as Madrid. There, it attracted the attention of moralists, hygienists and medical men who theorized about its causes and pronounced means by which it might be controlled. In his review of Spanish public health in 1884, Hauser voiced contemporary medical consensus in identifying alcoholism as a sickness that was so widespread that it was causing degeneration of the human race (*siglo* 209). He cites statistics culled throughout Europe documenting increased consumption of alcohol with parallel increase in alcoholism-related deaths. Like his peers in England and France, he attributes this trend to the "colossal" increase in industrial distillation of cheaper and more toxic spirits from starchy root crops at the expense of the traditional spirits derived from distillation of wine.[4] Hauser quotes further statistics from European and the United States showing increases in insanity and crime that were related to chronic intoxication. He notes in addition that in countries where military service was obligatory, the majority of recruits

3 The wide availability of cheap distilled spirits is universally deplored by contemporary writers including Huss, Morel and Hauser. Increasingly sophisticated distillation equipment followed advances in the knowledge of the physics of heat and the use of steam for heating such that not only could denser mixtures of grain and root crops be distilled, often after chemical treatment, but techniques permitting continuous distillation resulted in vastly increased efficiency in the output and concentration of alcohol. Many of these advances took place in France, though, "the most influential design of the period was that of Aeneas Coffey patented [in Britain] in 1830" (R.J.Forbes 348). An idea of the advances in technical sophistication of distillation in Spain can be had by comparing the text of Gutiérrez Bueno (1787) with those of Roura (1839) and Méndez and Pereda (1858).

4 The toxicologists Dujardin-Beaumetz and Audigé reported in 1878 that, in contrast with spirits distilled from wine that produced almost pure ethyl alcohol, spirits derived from root crops (sugar beet, potatoes) and grain contained quantities of butyl, propyl and amyl alcohols that were considered to be significantly more toxic (17). They comment that the spirits in Sweden, where chronic alcoholism was at "its greatest intensity" and was first described by Huss, were made from potatoes (18).

rejected by the armed services were either alcoholics or the children of alcoholics (*siglo* 211).

Citing the struggle for existence and the poor diet seen in "modern society" Hauser allies himself with degenerationist currents of thought in contemporary French alienist psychiatry. This rhetoric of degeneration was present in France at the beginning of the nineteenth century, though it had very ancient origins as a narrative to explain human ills. Drawing on that tradition,[5] the *aliéniste* Morel made it the cornerstone of his classification of mental disease to replace the monomania nosology (classification of disease) of his predecessor, Esquirol. Morel claimed that diseases resulting from the noxious effects of modern life lead to a degenerative fall from the natural state of biblical perfection.[6] Seeing many working-class patients from the nearby, harsh industrial suburbs of Rouen at the asylum of Sainte-Yon where he worked, he quickly identified the role of alcohol in the production of disease. In addition, he attributed to the process of degeneration crime, insanity and hereditary impairment extending to the fourth generation, leading to extinction of the family line.[7] Morel's pupil, Magnan, abandoned the idea of progressive degeneration from a state of biblical perfection in favour of the concept of retrograde degeneration to a more primitive state. This he attributes to inadequacy in the individual's

5 It has become popular to attribute the idea of degeneration to Morel, one author even claiming that he coined the term. In fact, the tradition of degenerationist thought goes back to Classical antiquity. Buffon published his essay *De la dégénération des animaux* in 1766, while both, *dégénération* and *dégénérescence*, appear frequently in Fodéré's *Traite de médecine légal …* of 1813. Savoyen published his *Nouvelles études philosophiques sur la dégénération physique et morale de l'homme* (1854) three years before Morel's first magnum opus. For fuller accounts of the genealogy of the concept, see the studies of Genil-Perrin, Bénichou, and Stannard (*Degeneration*).

6 "a pathological deviation from the normal type of humanity," "une déviation maladive du type normal de l'humanité" (*Dégénérescences* 74).

7 Dowbiggin 118. The idea of alcohol abuse leading to progressive, inherited degeneration ending in extinction appears in a footnote in Erasmus Darwin's *The Botanic Garden*, "It is remarkable that all the diseases from drinking spirituous or fermented liquors are liable to become hereditary, even to the third generation; gradually increasing, if the cause be continued, till the family becomes extinct" (*II The Loves of Plants*, 111).

struggle for survival in an increasingly stressful urban and industrial world.[8] Such a view clearly reflects the influence of Darwin's *On the Origin of Species* and its popularization by the writings of Herbert Spencer. As a physical influence associated with disease, crime, prostitution, insanity and damaged descendants, alcoholism became one of the cornerstones of Magnan's degenerationist psychiatric thinking for the rest of the nineteenth century.[9]

Alcoholism and public inebriation were seen to be associated not only with the ills of the individual in society but also with a potential for mass political agitation. Employers worried about diminished reliability and productivity of their workers. In an attempt to control the problem, temperance movements enjoyed some success, mostly in northern European countries. In Spain, however, where powerful commercial lobbies fought any legislation that might compromise their interests, the temperance movement achieved, effectively, nothing.[10] Galdós describes the unregulated saturation of one of Madrid's poorer districts with *tabernas* in *Fortunata y Jacinta*. As Guillermina and Jacinta journey down the *calle Toledo* to visit a tenement, *corral de vecindad*, of Madrid's poor, Jacinta exclaims on the presence of so many red-painted tavern doors:

> Oh! the red was so abundant that it seemed that the community's religion was that of blood […] The doors of the taverns were also the colour of blood. And they were not just one or two. Jacinta was alarmed to see so many, and Guillermina could only pronounce: "What perdition! One door a tavern and the next one not. All crime comes from here."[11]

8 Huertas García-Alejo 363.

9 Magnan (*l'alcoolisme*). Magnan's student, Paul Legrain (1860–1939), was responsible for a related text *Dégénéscence sociale y alcoolisme* in 1895, the same year in which both co-authored *Les dégénérés*.

10 Cervera Barat 161; Campos, *Alcoholismo* 231–32.

11 "¡Oh!, el rojo abundaba tanto, que aquello parecía un pueblo que tiene la religión de la sangre. […] Las puertas de las tabernas también de color de sangre. Y que no son ni una ni dos. Jacinta se asustaba de ver tantas, y Guillermina no pudo menos de exclamar: '¡Cuánta perdición!, una puerta sí y otra no, taberna. De aquí salen todos los crímenes'" (*Fortunata I* 318).

While drunkenness had been recorded since biblical times and was traditionally regarded as a vice,[12] the condition began to receive closer attention of physicians in the early nineteenth century and, as a consequence, became progressively medicalized. A detailed description of drunkenness was published by Thomas Trotter in 1804, while the tremor, hallucinations and mania that follow interruption of prolonged alcohol intake, *delirium tremens*, received its first detailed description by Thomas Sutton in 1813. Only in 1849, however, was chronic alcoholism defined as a specific disease entity as a result of the work of the Swede, Magnus Huss (1807–90). The value of his publication, in which he coined the term *alcoholismus chronicos*, was immediately recognized in France where a translation and commentary were provided by Renaudin. Huss was also influential in the work of Morel (*Dégénérescences* 369–70), and is cited in Spanish texts such as those of Giné y Partagas (*freno-patología* 462–63) and the translation from the French of Jaccoud (*III* 783 ff.).

In fiction, detailed description of alcoholism is a hallmark of the Naturalistic writings of Émile Zola, whose novel *l'Assommoir* (1877) explores it in unsparing detail. Galdós's first novel in this new genre, *La desheredada* (1881), was originally drafted to include a number of scenes illustrating the destructive influence of drink. However, they were expunged from the published version, together with other more brutal portrayals, possibly to avoid too close a similarity with Zola's work.[13] An attenuated scene of intoxication that remains is at the end of the novel where Isidora's pathetic champion, José Relimpio, dies gently after being faced with the reality of his godchild's determination to abandon herself to the streets.

Medical texts of the day recognized three more or less similar degrees of acute inebriation.[14] The first level was that of "agreeable excitement" and a feeling of expansive well-being, the second was that of "disordered

12 Bynum, 161.

13 Schnepf's study of the early manuscript version of *La desheredada* reveals that *la Sanguijuelera* is brutalized by *aguardiente* in part of a "tirade against taverns and drinking" (58).

14 Giné y Partagas, *freno-patología* 464, Jaccoud 280–82, Lancereaux 5–7, Pulido, *Bosquejos* 233–35, Renaudin (Huss) 65–66, Santero 367.

excitement" with disturbed thought processes and lack of judgement in which, "the subject becomes so talkative that he reveals things that he would be better advised to keep quiet about, hence the expression *in vino veritas*."[15] Authorities concur that further drinking beyond this point leads to the third stage characterized by prostration, coma and even death.

In *Fortunata y Jacinta*, Galdós portrays differing levels of intoxication that cast characterizing light upon three figures of the story. The first involves Juanito Santa Cruz in a lapse from bourgeois decorum on his honeymoon with Jacinta, when he allows himself to be bullied into over-indulgence by a drunk Englishman at a wedding reception in their *fonda* in Triana.[16] Unguardedly loquacious, he praises the physical charms of his former mistress, Fortunata, and reveals details of his affair that his bride had been trying to glean from him. He admits the heartlessness of his deception of Fortunata and mocks her guilelessness that enabled him to seduce and then abandon her. Absorbed in self-pity and remorse, he begs Jacinta's forgiveness at the same time that he recounts details of his violent break with the pregnant Fortunata and his readiness to strike her protector and uncle, José Izquerdo, to the ground. This portrayal of the second stage of acute inebriation in Juanito occurs in the context of the privileged upper middle-class for whom drunkenness was a disgraceful lapse of self-control. There is no other such episode that involves Juanito in the novel and we can regard it as an isolated, though highly revealing, one.

In contrast with the exceptional episode of acute drunkenness of Juanito, Galdós includes in the story of *Fortunata y Jacinta* a portrait of habitual drunkenness in the figure of José Izquerdo, which falls within the category of chronic alcoholism defined by Magnus Huss. We are

15 "el hombre se hace tan comunicativo, que revela lo que racionalmente debiera callarse, por eso se ha dicho *in vino veritas*" (Giné y Partagas, *freno-patología* 464, author's italics).

16 *Fortunata I* 225 ff. Bourgeois pretentions to sobriety in comparison with the lower orders are vividly illustrated by the profound sense of shame that haunts Ido de Sagrario elsewhere in the novel when a relative succeeds in getting him drunk for the only time in his life, "the memory of the degradation of that night saddened him every time he recalled it," "el recuerdo de la degradación de aquella noche le entristecía siempre que repuntaba en su memoria" (*Fortunata I* 175).

memorably introduced to his life history, which we later discover is entirely fictional, when he cadges a meal from the teetotal José Ido de Sagrario. He impresses the latter with his great tolerance for drink, "[José Izquierdo] drained his glass once again, and the other José found his eloquence and his capacity for drink equally remarkable."[17] In the course of the novel, Izquierdo is shown to be a lazy and ineffectual imposter who is easily cowed by Guillermina Pacheco when she penetrates his bluster in order to beat down the price in her bargaining for the false *Pitusín* (*Fortunata I* 368 ff.). We also see him repeatedly in the closing chapters of the story where he is ordering or consuming quantities of beer drinking himself into a stupor. While his habitual tipple appears to be beer, he is also reported to be able to drink *aguardiente* like water.[18]

Society at this time often failed to distinguish between drinking, drunkenness and alcoholism, and temperance reformers in northern European countries maintained that drinking invariably led to drunkenness (Harrison 21). At the same time, however, it was recognized that individuals' tolerance for drink was not equal and that some drinkers seemed to be able to "hold their drink" better than others.[19] What was very clear was that it varied with the variety of alcoholic drink consumed. Intermittent drunkenness due to consumption of wine and beer was seen as being more or less sustainable in many individuals. A regime of distilled spirits such as *aguardiente*, however, was recognised to be more damaging and more prone to lead to chronic alcoholism.

17 "[Izquierdo] Apuró de nuevo el vaso, y el otro José admiraba igualmente su facundia y su receptividad de bebedor" (*Fortunata I* 343).

18 "y su amigo Izquierdo, que bebía aguardiente como si fuera agua" (*Fortunata II* 425).

19 Lancereaux refers to variation in the effects of alcohol including, "des dispositions particulières des individus" (*l'alcoolisme* 5), while Renaudin emphasizes, "l'idiosynchrasie individuelle" (64). A paragraph from a text in Galdós's library also makes the point, "individual predisposition has a very well-established influence, since not all drinkers become chronic alcoholics even, if they consume the same quantity of alcohol," "La predisposición individual tiene una influencia positive bien demostrada, porque no todos los bebedores, aunque consuman igual cantidad de bebida, llegan á alcoholizarse" (Jaccoud *III* 780).

An unforgettable depiction of chronic alcohol dependence in *Fortunata y Jacinta* occurs in the character of Mauricia la Dura. She first makes her appearance in the convent of las Micaelas, which is partly devoted to reforming wayward women with a view to returning them to respectable society. She has been referred there by Guillermana Pacheco, the *santa fundadora*, with a view to correcting her drunkenness and intermittent prostitution.

Mauricia immediately recognizes Fortunata as a previous fellow employee of the brothel of *la Paca* where Juanito, Fortunata's lover, had been a client. Fortunata develops a close rapport with Mauricia with her, "puzzling alternations of depravity and good nature."[20] The narrator describes Mauricia's unpredictable attacks of fury, the first of which fills Fortunata with terror. Using foul language and physical menaces, Mauricia appears to hold the sisters of the convent and the other women to be reformed, the *recoletas*, at her will until the dwarfed, limping nun, Sor Marcela, exercises a calming influence over her and escorts her to a room where she can be confined for the night.

From the window of her cell, Mauricia watches her captor go about her duties in the convent garden. With her fury completely extinguished, she implores a little of Sor Marcela's cache of cognac, "bring me just a little [tear] drop of that divine glory that you keep."[21] Galdós's picture of a wild woman reduced to infantile cajoling is a vivid picture of the intensity of the craving of the chronic alcoholic. At first ignoring her pleas, Marcela later brings her an evening meal and then measures out for her a small quantity of cognac, which results in a show of extreme gratitude and temporarily reformed behaviour from Mauricia. The narrator explains the humane reasoning behind Marcela's actions, "absolute deprivation of appetites fed by more or less depraved habits is the worst of remedies since it results

20 "alternativas misterios de depravación y afabilidad" (*Fortunata I* 608).

21 "Tráeme nada más que una lagrimita de aquella gloria divina que tú tienes" (*Fortunata I* 615–16).

in despair, and it is advisable to indulge [those appetites] very cautiously now and again."[22]

Galdós here touches on the thorny problem of how chronic alcoholics should best be managed, which had divided authorities since the beginning of the century. Long before Huss defined the disease, some physicians recommended complete abstinence as the only effective path to cure. Others, however, chose the apparently more humane path of permitting small doses of alcohol in order to ward off the worst of withdrawal symptoms which, at their most acute, produced *delirium tremens*. Galdós has Sor Marcela adopt the latter course, showing later in the narrative how ineffective it is in Mauricia's case. Interestingly, opinion on treatment seems to have been divided on English-Continental lines according to Bynum:

> The goal of his [Trotter's] therapy (and that of many of his English contemporaries) was complete abstinence. This contrasts strikingly with the situation on the Continent, where moderation was the goal of physicians treating alcoholism in the first half of the 19th century. Only with the efforts of the psychiatrists Forel, Kraepelin, and their fellow workers did abstinence become the ultimate goal in the treatment of alcoholism in Continental Europe.[23]

Mauricia's ultimately tragic story suggests that Galdós, either from personal observation or from what he learned from other sources, may in this respect have been ahead of the consensus of Spanish medicine of his time.

Galdós's vividly realistic account of Mauricia's lapse into *locura alcohólica* in *Las Micaelas* strongly suggests that he had observed similar frightening behaviour at firsthand. The features of his portrait can also be found, however, in descriptions such as that of Giné y Partagas, written ten years before *Fortunata y Jacinta* was composed. After seeming to behave in a controlled manner, Mauricia helps Fortunata hunt throughout Sor Marcela's cell for a mouse that is terrifying the nun, and succeeds in

22 "… la privación absoluta de los apetitos alimentados por la costumbre más o menos viciosa, es el peor de los remedios, por engendrar la desesperación, y que para curar añejos defectos es conveniente permitirlos de vez en cuando con mucha medida" (*Fortunata I* 621).

23 Bynum 168.

capturing and dispatching it (*I* 636). Soon afterwards, however, she is found weeping in a state of acute remorse. A mood change is then revealed by repressed laughter and a satanic smile, which Fortunata cannot understand (*I* 639). When the convent school pupils, the *Josefinas*, retreat from the heat of the day to the convent garden, Mauricia appears withdrawn, later confessing to a fellow detainee that she has seen the Virgin Mary (*I* 641). She describes the Virgin as weeping as she walked in the garden without her Son, and seeing many little angels about the garden tree. At first muttering incoherently to herself, she then rises like one inspired announcing, "Oh my Lady! I will bring him to you, I will bring him to you,"[24] only to retire to bed where Fortunata takes her to be deeply asleep. However, she rises later and, when unable to enter the chapel whose door is locked, collapses into a deep sleep in which she dreams that she is able to make an entry. In her dream, she walks to the altar which she climbs in order to remove the monstrance containing the Host, which bears human features, and which she hears protesting at its removal (*I* 647).

Next morning she is found sitting, withdrawn, on a pile of manure in the orchard unresponsive to calls to join the others. Despite all the talk of visions, the Mother Superior seems to realize that things are not to be accounted for by the purely religious and recommends that a doctor be called (*I* 650). At this point Sor Marcela appears with an empty cognac bottle, realizing that Mauricia must have drained it during the search for the mouse in her cell. Attempts to restrain Mauricia are met by invective and a hail of stones and manure causing terror throughout the convent. She is finally subdued by blows from the chaplain and is thrown, half-dressed, into the street. There, giving and receiving a torrent of abuse from the crowd, she is followed by a band of mocking youths as she walks away from the convent.

One reads this scene as one might an account of an out-of-control patient in an asylum, so seemingly authentic are Mauricia's symptoms and her unreasoning, self-defeating rage. In a masterly stoke, Galdós has Mauricia dream that she restores Christ to his forlorn mother hinting that she may have been acting out her own feelings about the loss of custody of

24 "¡Oh mi señora! ... Te lo traeré, te lo traeré" (*Fortunata I* 644).

her own daughter, Adoración. He describes attempts of the religious community to understand what is happening to their rebellious fellow inmate. We can find the three main elements that Galdós incorporates into his description, depression, mania, and hallucinating psychosis, listed by Giné y Partagas in his description of alcoholic madness. Giné describes acute alcoholic mania, a state of violent agitation that is associated with vivid hallucinations and distorted thought. He describes *melancolía alcohólica*, second to mania in frequency, also associated with hallucination. Giné has difficulty in distinguishing the most advanced form of alcoholic insanity from insanity arising from other causes that are made worse by alcohol, citing its association with paranoia. In his time, there was uncertainty about the nature of the dementia in which chronic alcoholism could terminate, and its relation to tertiary, syphilitic G.P.I. Attempting to distinguish between the two, Giné quotes Fournier's table comparing the two conditions, only to conclude that they might be indistinguishable.[25] Giné glumly concludes by observing that once the features of chronic alcoholism had made their appearance, the condition was likely to be incurable (*freno-patología* 475–76). This assessment appears to be shared by Galdós for, after several episode of scandalous public intoxication, the severely ill Mauricia is finally moved to the home of her sister, Severiana, for what proves to be terminal care. In his separate description of *locura alcoholica*, Santero adds the, "irresistible desire to break and destroy everything," something that the good Protestant missionaries, Horacio and Malvina, are shown

25 Giné y Partagas lists features that could be used to distinguish *locura alcoholica* from G.P.I. that he attributes to Alfred Fournier of France (*freno-patología* 472–73). This, however, was problematic since many patients with alcoholism probably had G.P.I., and there was no way at the time to confirm the presence of syphilitic infection. In 1883, Giné observed to Seguin that, in his experience, chronic alcoholism was a common predisposing cause of the much-increased incidence of G.P.I. (412). The reliance of Giné and other Spanish writers on descriptions of alcoholism by French authors is striking. Campos notes of Spain of the time, "the absence of original investigative work about the effects of alcohol" and the, "scientific dependence upon foreign sources, notably the French," "la inexistencia de trabajos originales de investigación sobre los efectos del alcohol" and the, "dependencia científica de la producción foránea, en especial francesa" (*Alcoholismo* 37).

to discover to their cost when Mauricia destroys the furnishings of their chapel (*II* 167).[26]

Galdós's fascination for the processes of dying is well-known and, in the case of Mauricia, he does not spare medical detail.[27] We learn that in her delirium, she has attacked both Guillermina and the Protestants who were trying to help her, and that after being discharged from Hospital for a third time, at Guillermina's request, she has been sent to the home of her sister, Severiana, for terminal care.

It has been observed that the alcoholism of José Izquierdo and Mauricia la Dura is portrayed very differently, since the latter's acute episodes of intoxication in public were considered more scandalous by contemporaries than the more private inebriation of Izquierdo.[28] Public drunkenness in women, the supposed guardians of the morality of the home and promoters of domestic values to be passed on to children, was less tolerated by *madrileños* than street inebriation in men.[29] Galdós has been interpreted as portraying this double standard consistent with the male-dominated outlook of the bourgeois of his time. In contrast with this, however, it might be argued that Izquierdo's alcoholism is not truly comparable to Mauricia's. Not only does don José seem to restrict his drinking to taverns

26 "The acute mania of drinkers [...] is characterized by an irresistible tendency to break and destroy everything," "La manía aguda de los bebedores [...] está caracterizada por un irresistible propensión á romperlo todo y á destruirlo" (Santero 373).

27 Montesinos observes, "Galdós [...] does not allow anyone to die without listening [to their chest] and taking their pulse, nor does he fail to detail their symptoms, or spare medical jargon," "(Galdós [...] no deja ya morir a nadie sin auscultarlo y tomarle el pulso, ni deja de puntualizar los síntomas, sin ahorrar tecnicismos)" (*II* 88).

28 Fuentes Peris 87–109.

29 In the context of damage to the family by drunkenness, Concepción Arenal writes, "The damage is even greater when the mother provides the bad example or follows it, and, treading on duty and honour, joins her husband in filthy excesses, and in the storm of such excesses does not even extend to her children that plank of salvation that is called *my mother's virtue*," "El daño es todavía mayor cuando la mujer da el mal ejemplo ó le sigue, y hollando deber y honor, acompaña á su marido á las inmundas orgías, y en la borrasca de tantos excesos ni aun deja á los hijos aquella tabla de salvación que se llama *la virtud de mi madre*" (*Pauperismo*, 292, author's italics).

and the home, but he habitually intersperses his *aguardiente* consumption with large quantities of beer. In addition to the long-recognized wide variation of individual tolerance of alcohol that was recorded in medical texts of the time was the observation that though chronic alcoholism was more commonly seen in men, its effects were more serious in women.[30] While the end result of his addiction may be the same over time, Izquierdo's poisoning with a variety of alcoholic drinks appears to be less medically and socially damaging than Mauricia's uniform preference for distilled spirits. Izquierdo may be on the way to the later stages of the *alcoholismus chronicus* that Magnus Huss describes, but Mauricia, as her demise in *delirium tremens* later confirms, has already long arrived.

The descriptions of Mauricia's outrageous behaviour reveal much about contemporary ambivalence about the way that her condition should be viewed. doña Lupe, Nicolás and the narrator all appear to conform to the traditional view when they refer to her condition as being one of a bad habit or *vicio*, implying that it is something amenable to moral persuasion. This explanation is seen to exist side by side with a medical interpretation, inherited from authorities like Trotter, Sutton and Huss, that regards alcoholism as a sickness for which referral to a physician or hospital is necessary. For not only does the Mother Superior at *Las Micaelas* call for a doctor, but Mauricia is repeatedly admitted to hospital for treatment and, when discharged, is seen at home by the doctor of the *Beneficencia Domiciliaria* and *Junta de señoras*.[31] The view of Mauricia's *delirium tremens as* organic in nature appears to be confirmed by Galdós when he has the unnamed doctor prescribe *nux vomica* and morphine to control her delirium, as well as regular quantities of sherry.[32]

30 Renaudin's précis of Huss's work contains the observation, "One observes [alcoholism] above all in men, but it has the gravest effects on women," "On l'observe surtout chez les hommes, mais il a des consequences plus graves chez les femmes" (86). It is possible that Galdós also observed this.

31 "the home welfare doctor of the Ladies' Committee was visiting her," "la asistía el médico de la Beneficencia Domiciliaria y de la Junta de señoras" (*Fortunata II* 171)

32 *Nux vomica* is derived from strychnine. Together with opiates and sherry, *Nux vomica* was recommended in the treatment of *delirium tremens* by Jaccoud in Galdós's edition of the *Tratado*. Jaccoud quotes Magnus Huss as authority for the practice.

The issue of conflicting explanatory narratives is a complex one since many physicians of the time also continued to adhere to the alcoholism-as-vice perspective. Like their hygienist colleagues, they tended to view alcoholism as a vice typical of the labouring classes and, as such, the root cause of their improvident misery. It has been suggested by historians such as Campos, that the bourgeois took advantage of the label of alcoholism as an explanation for a whole range of social problems that underlay the much debated issue of urban poverty, the *cuestión social*. The argument ran that urban poverty was a self-inflicted vice, and that the lower orders were responsible for their own plight.[33] Such a view, of course, had the advantage of relieving the middle classes of any sense of responsibility for improving the environmental conditions of the poor or for working to improve social justice. At the same time, alcoholism was seen by hygienists, as living proof of the reality of degeneration at work, with its narrative of inherited predisposition to alcoholism and a related cluster of conditions such as madness, crime, prostitution and national decline.[34] All these conditions were seen as contributing to social and political instability. For practical purposes, it seems that the poverty of others was something that the urban well-to-do could live with; the prospect of social instability and a change in the *status quo*, however, was something that had to be taken more seriously.

In the course of his description of Mauricia's final illness, Galdós accumulates for us much clinical information, revealing his study of chronic alcoholism. He tells us that Mauricia is running a fever and that she has lost her appetite, in addition to developing the tremor of limbs and face characteristic of *delirium tremens*. He gives her an epileptic convulsion, a feature to be found in contemporary descriptions. In contrast with some authorities who regarded the condition as being comparable to intoxication with poisons, he is aware that the precipitating event in *delirium tremens* is, in fact, the sudden withdrawal of alcohol to which the nervous system has become habituated. Such is the hallmark of addiction and contrasts

33 Campos Marín, *vicio* 284, Campos Marín, *Alcoholismo* 38 ff.; 99 ff., Campos Marín and Huertas García-Alejo 264–72.

34 This the theme of Cervera Barat in his *Alcoholismo y civilización*.

with heavy-metal intoxication with poisons like mercury, copper and lead with which Renaudin (Huss) compare it (84). He understands the paradox of treating the addicted patient with measured quantities of alcohol, a counter-intuitive treatment obviously known to Mauricia's anonymous physician but scandalizing Severiana and doña Lupe to whom it looks like fanning the flames of the disease. Galdós has the shrewd and down-to-earth doña Lupe express surprise that the patient should be treated with regular quantities of sherry, which she knows contains the alcohol responsible for Mauricia's parlous state, "but are you really giving her ... that perdition?" to which Severiana answers, "the doctor has ordered it. He says that it is medicine. It seems to me to be the reverse, I can tell you."[35]

The apparently incidental descriptions of Mauricia contain many features that appear in medical texts. We are told from the beginning of her hoarse voice, *ronca*, associated at that time with drinking. In her last phases, Galdós not only makes her suffer from breathlessness but also adds the description of a cavernous voice that "seemed to come from the depth of a deep pitcher and sounded very distant."[36] Both features are described in Galdós's edition of Jaccoud (*III* 788).

More clinical detail is to come, however, as we are informed that the doctor examines Maurica carefully and finds that her abdomen and legs are swollen and that her *parálisis agitante* is much worse. For those of his readers uncertain of the significance of the abnormally big abdomen, Galdós explains it in an indirect fashion by having Guillermina describe a

35 "¿Pero de veras le dais ... esa perdición? – preguntó alarmadísima doña Lupe. – Lo ha mandado el médico. Dice que es medicina. Parece aquello de *al revés te lo digo*" (*Fortunata II* 176, author's italics). There was a marked difference between the treatment of *delirium tremens* depending upon whether a cure was being attempted or whether palliation in terminal care was being undertaken. While Huss maintains that withdrawal of all alcohol is a necessary treatment if a cure is to be effected (Renaudin 68), Galdós's copy of Jaccoud quotes the Swedish authority as recommending the "moderate use of port or sherry" to control severe *delirium* when other medications fail (*III* 800). Clearly in Mauricia's case, where cure is not being attempted, any measure to reduce the agonies of withdrawal is considered appropriate.

36 "su voz parecía salir del hueco de un cántaro muy hondo, y sonaba como lejos" (*Fortunata II* 224).

neighbour with a similar case of hydropsy and a huge abdomen. She relates that three attempts to tap the fluid obtained only half a litre of free fluid whereas the size of the abdomen suggested that it must have contained about 14 litres. Fluid swelling of the lower limbs and accumulation of fluid within the abdomen (*ascites*) are described in Jaccoud (*III* 20–21) and were understood to be associated with scarring of the liver, cirrhosis (62), which was known to occur in chronic alcoholism (57). Loss of weight together with swelling of the lower limbs was observed by Huss (Renaudin 69). The basic observations of terminal liver failure seen in end-stage chronic alcoholism were thus circulating in medical texts at the time that Galdós wrote. What is remarkable is that he was sufficiently interested in the clinical details to incorporate so many of them, entirely appropriately, into his moving depiction of Mauricia's end.[37]

The theme of alcoholism also appears frequently in *Ángel Guerra* among its many portrayals of disease and deformity. In don Pito, Galdós creates the figure of a retired sailor, a genial rogue with a longstanding, daily need for alcoholic spirits. Like Izquierdo, he frequently drinks himself into a stupor without, apparently, developing the florid mental disturbance and liver failure that mark Mauricia's decline.

An alcohol dependence of relatively low-profile recurs in the minor character, the miscast-by-life priest Eleuterio Virones, who is happier working on constructions projects at the villas, *cigarrales*, of Gauadalupe and Turleque than attending to more meditative matters. Perhaps coincidentally, contemporaries also observed a greater tolerance for alcohol in men involved in hard physical labour. By contrast, the figure of Dulcenombre, drowning the shock of her rejection by Guerra in the *ponche* she is introduced to by

37 That Mauricia should die with the savour of sherry on her lips is consistent with the medical practice of the day. That witnesses should disagree about the significance of her dying words (Lupe thought she was calling for more sherry rather than beholding the glory of the afterlife) is a feature of Galdós's fondness for ambiguity in such matters and recalls the dying utterance of Torquemada in *Torquemada y San Pedro*. Also, as Galdós was a great admirer of Shakespeare, it may not be a coincidence that Nym and the Hostess agreed that a call for sherry was on the dying lips of that other larger-than-life character, Falstaff.

don Pito, is an interesting intermediate between acute and chronic alcoholism, since she becomes habituated to drink without developing *delirium tremens*. Her shocking diatribe as a result of her rejection (385) offends her mother doña Catalina as much as it does Guerra for its incompatibility with the standards of accepted womanly behaviour, but is perfectly understandable in her situation. She lacks the psychotic hallucinations that afflict Mauricia.

The priest, don Juan Casado employs the social-religious (alcoholism as vice) perspective on alcohol dependence with persuasive warnings and witty parables, "con persuasivas amonestaciones y chuscas parabolas" (436) without success. At this point Galdós's anonymous *médico* employs the medical (alcoholism as disease) approach by allowing her limited and very carefully measured quantities of spirits.[38] In this he appears to be conforming to Sor Marcela's "Continental" therapeutic approach where Dulce's withdrawal symptoms are made more bearable while she is sedated. A close reading of the text, however, raises the question that Galdós may have known in unsuspected detail about a variety of treatment for alcoholism. We are informed that the *médico* prescribed medications with an alcoholic base as a result of which Dulce developed such a strong distaste for drink that she vomited, even at the smell of alcohol. Such a sequence of events suggests that the *médico* may have prescribed a medication causing nausea in her alcohol-based medicine so as to produce a powerful aversion.[39]

In contrast again, don Pito is a confirmed chronic alcoholic for whom abstinence is impossible. Ángel exhorts him at the end of the novel not in order that he give up drink, but that he maintain a respectably low profile in his drunkenness, "emborracharse decorosamente" (686). As Ángel is dying and disposes of his estate, he bequeaths Pito a perpetual drink allowance, implicitly acknowledging that he is completely beyond cure (715), a victim of chronic alcoholism whose date with *delirium tremens* has yet to fall due.

38 "La enferma tomó [bebidas espirituosas] con gusto porciones muy tasadas" (*Guerra* 436).

39 Aversion therapy for alcoholism is thus not new. Since the 1920s, the drug *Antabuse* has been used to help treat alcoholics by making them feel nauseated every time they taste alcohol.

CHAPTER 5

Madness

Galdós's fondness for portraying characters with altered mental states as well as overt lunacy has been repeatedly observed. From his early *La novela en el tranvía* and *La sombra* (1871) and throughout his *Novelas contemporáneas* (1881–89) depictions of madness occur together with those of obsession, and a variety of eccentricities bordering on madness. While Galdós seems to anticipate the focus on abnormal and marginal behaviour, which became even more evident in the literature of the 1890s, Baroja saw it as part of a tradition of modern, as opposed to classical, writing, "modern heroes, from Don Quijote and Hamlet to Raskolnikov, are inspired and mad. All great modern literature is created on the basis of mental disturbance."[1] Galdós's interest in variations of mental incapacity extends to the grotesquely abnormal, exemplified by the *monstruo*, Juan, in *Ángel Guerra* and the wretchedly retarded second Valentín in the last two *Torquemada* novels.[2] Consistent with the understanding of his time, Galdós makes the grotesquely retarded characters close relatives of genius-prodigies (Sabas and Valentín I), themselves regarded as varieties of madness.[3] His portrayals reveal an overlap

1 "los héroes modernos, desde Don Quijote y Hamlet hasta Raskólnikov, son inspirados y locos. Toda la gran literatura moderna está hecha a base de perturbaciones mentales" (*Desde* 439).

2 *Torquemada en el purgatorio* (1894) and *Torquemada y San Pedro* (1895).

3 A close hereditary relationship between genius and insanity/imbecility was suggested in 1859 by Jacques-Joseph Moreau de Tours (1804–84), and became a widely held view in the later nineteenth century, "the hereditary correlation of the two most extreme conditions in which the human spirit can find itself, madness and the most elevated intellectual abilities," "la corrélation héréditaire des deux conditions les plus extremes dans lesquelles l'esprit humain puisse se trouver la folie et les aptitudes les

between mental abnormality and the grotesque, the latter a well-recognized tradition in Spanish letters (Nimitz 135–36, Kronik 39–40).

So numerous are Galdós's mentally disturbed characters that an analysis of them all would require a text on that topic alone. What follows is a selection of figures that demonstrates Galdós's awareness of contemporary thinking on mental disease in Spain and its debt to the dominant ideas of the pre-Freudian psychiatry of that time (*alienism*), which originated in France.

One of Galdós most celebrated depictions of madness is that of Tomás Rufete in the opening chapter of *La desheredada*. From the first line of the novel, we are immersed in the details of a hallucinating mania of an inmate of Madrid's public asylum of *Santa Isabel de Leganés*. Rufete believes himself to have responsibility for high financial matters in the Spanish state and is obsessed with huge sums of money that are impossible to control, "Oh [enormous] sum as trembling, elusive and ungraspable as a drop of mercury!"[4] The raving patient is approached by a physician (serious, *serio*, and kind, *bondadoso*, are adjectives of the kind that Galdós commonly uses to describe physicians in the exercise of their art), who prescribes a double dose of the sedative potassium bromide in an attempt to calm him.[5]

---

plus élevées de l'intelligence" (385). Later development of the idea is described by Huertas (*Madness*).

4 "¡oh cantidad temblorosa, escurridiza, inaprensible, como una gota de mercurio" (67–68). Citations of *La desheredada* are from the Cátedra edition edited by Germán Gullón hereafter cited as *desheredada*.

5 Potassium bromide was introduced into therapeutics after a medical meeting in London in 1857 when Sir Charles Locock reported his experience in its use as a remedy for hysteria in young women, having read of its use to diminish sexual drive. He also found it very effective in the treatment of "hysterical epilepsy" related to menstruation (528). It was endorsed more scientifically by Sir Samuel Wilks in 1861 (Eadie 276). Convulsions were commonly attributed at the time to masturbation, and bromide was at first thought to act by reducing sexual arousal. It was later widely employed as a sedative and remained the only effective anticonvulsant until the introduction of Phenobarbital in 1912 (Scott 114). Giné y Partagas in 1876 records daily use of high-dose potassium bromide as a sedative in his asylum (*freno-patología* 277).

The sedation appears to be ineffective, however, since Rufete proceeds to harangue a tree trunk with his fiscal woes. When the physician returns and tries to reason with him, he obstinately adheres to the idea of mercury in his head and his urgent need to attend to matters of the *Congreso*. He is then transferred to the poorest accommodation in the asylum as a result of no maintenance payments for him having been received by the hospital. There, he habitually avoids the burly and unsympathetic asylum warders, seeing them as the sworn enemies of his high political aims, and as the souls of envy (73). He continues to address an imaginary crowd of high officials that depend upon the authorization of his signature. He also conducts long conversations with the water tumbling from a fountain. One day, however, he becomes withdrawn and silent and, on being taken to the asylum hospital, is prescribed a cold shower treatment, "the water torture," *la inquisición de agua* (77). Rufete is familiar with this brutal procedure and struggles ineffectively to escape it, as he is tied to an iron ring attached to the wall. He is exhausted by the "treatment" and the next that we hear of him is that he has died (90).

Galdós visited the asylum of Leganés several times to research the details for this chapter and its portrait of Tomás Rufete. His description indicates the care with which he studied the symptoms and treatment of the mad. In addition to portraying the manifestations of mania, Galdós also brilliantly uses Rufete's ravings to make pertinent criticisms of the Spanish fiscal establishment. At the same time, he provides a moving critique of the crowding and inhumane conditions suffered by the inmates of what was supposedly Spain's model institution for the insane.[6]

6 The nightmarish conditions that Galdós describes in the Leganés asylum may have been accepted uncritically by some commentators. Villasante and Huertas have compared descriptions of foreign visitors such as Jelly and Seguin, which are not nearly as damning as Galdós's account, while the rival institution at Carabanchel Alto had many shortcomings that were less publicized. It is possible that Tolosa Latour's loyalty to Esquerdo and his institutions may have caused him to influence Galdós in his adverse description of Leganés. Tolosa published the first (Leganés) chapter of *La desheredada* in the short-lived *Diario médico* for which he wrote (Schmidt 29), making a powerful complementary contribution to the praises that he and Pulido heaped

The psychiatric profession in Spain had barely established itself at the time that Galdós wrote and many physicians responsible for asylum patients had no special training in the field. There was no coherent diagnostic or therapeutic narrative in the care of the insane for whom, in truth, therapeutic resources were extremely limited. Ideas about the causes and classification of mental disease were a jumble of different theories, largely imported from France, while the traditional religious view of insanity as sickness of the soul to be treated by religious means persisted in Spain.[7] Older physical measures such as purges and blood-letting were gradually replaced by varieties of psychological treatment that attempted to act upon the mind and emotions of the patient. This so-called *moral treatment*, in conjunction with the recommendation of non-restraint and the abolition of strait-jackets and manacles, was popularized in France as a result of the influence of Pinel.[8] In about 1810, in response to Pinels's perceived nosological shortcomings, his pupil Esquirol promulgated a new classification of

upon Esquerdo's asylums in the press in 1882. (Villasante, *instituciones* 83; Villasante and Huertas 29–30). Tolosa wrote a separate flattering portrait of Esquerdo for *El Imparcial* in 1880, while Pulido praised the opening of the Carabanchel asylum in 1877 attended, so he writes, by, "the cream of Madrid's medical profession," "la mayoría de las reputaciones médicas de Madrid," in the medical press (*Nuevo manicomio*). Tolosa managed to insert other good words about Esquerdo in his *Protección médica al niño desvalido* in 1881 (29), and at his *Discurso* before the *Congreso internacional para la protección de la infancia* in 1883 (15).

7 Esquerdo pours scorn on the metaphysical approach to mental illness, "those who belong to this [metaphysical] school resemble those who, having lost a needle look for it in the roof rather than on the floor [...] have to employ faith in these high and unknown regions for the investigation of mental illness [...] Happily we do not waste time in idle discussions today; [...] because all of us consider madness as an illness of the body," "los que pertenecen á esta escuela [metafísica] se semejan al que, habiendo perdido un alfiler, mirase al techo en vez de buscarle por el suelo [...] han de valarse de la fe para la exploración del trastorno en esas elevadas é ignotas regiones [...] Felizmente hoy no malversamos el tiempo en discusiones ociosas; [...] porque todos [...] consideran la locura enfermedad del cuerpo" (*Conferencias* 175). The lawyer and criminologist Dorado Montero (1861–1919) continued into the 1890s to view the criminal as suffering from a sickness of the soul (Campos and Huertas, *Lombroso* 314).

8 Pinel's achievements are discussed by Goldstein (chapter 3).

mental disease based upon the concept of *monomanía*, which became so influential that it accounted for 45% of diagnoses in a major psychiatric institution between the years 1826–33.[9] Many varieties of monomania were described, of which the modern usages of dipsomania, nymphomania and pyromania still survive. Esquirol's sucessors, Morel and Jean-Pierre Falret (1794–1870), in turn, worked hard to discredit monomania as a nosological entity with such success that it had disappeared as a diagnostic category at the Salpêtrière Hospital by 1870 (Goldstein, 152). In its place, Morel popularized a different classification of mental disease, based not on symptoms but on postulated causes, employing the ancient concept of degeneration. His work, and that of his successors Magnan and Legrain, ensured that the degenerationist account of mental disease, as well as a wide range of other social problems, remained the dominant discourse among *aliénistes* in France for the remainder of the nineteenth century. In contrast in the 1880s, Spanish *alienistas* continued to use the term *monomanía* freely, partly guided by texts such as the Spanish translation of Guislain's *Lecciones orales sobre las frenopatías* (1881), where it often appears (Stannard, *Degeneration* 21 n. 40). Pinel's enduring influence can be seen in the use of the term, *tratamiento moral*, in a text of Spain's leading *alienista* of the period, Giné y Partagas (*freno-patología* 264–66, 459).

The coexistence in Spain of religious interpretations of mental disease together with concepts inherited from Pinel, Esquirol and Morel resulted in a nosological free-for-all that leads one Spanish medical historian to refer to as a "hotchpotch," *mezcolanza*, the complex of concepts that coexisted in Spanish *alienismo*.[10] An advantage of this, from Galdós's point of view, was that he had a wide medical and conceptual vocabulary to draw upon in his portraits of the deranged.

9 Goldstein, 154.

10 "Concepts such as monomanía, neurosis, degeneration etc. follow each other in cascades, which provide a sample of the complex hotchpotch of concepts that still coexisted in Spanish psychiatry," "Conceptos como monomanía, neurosis, degeneración etc. se suceden en cascada, los que podría ser una muestra de la compleja mezcolanza conceptual que convivía todavía en la psiquiatría española" (Campos Marín, *Criminalidad* 117).

The depiction of Tomás Rufete, with his obsession with financial affairs of state and the impossibility of keeping track of huge sums of money, is combined with a description of vivid hallucinations that cause him to address imaginary, senior politicians. Galdós and his contemporaries could find just such a clinical picture described by Giné y Partagas as, "sensory or hallucinating monomanias-when the delirium of ideas, without being diffuse, but being circumscribed in a more or less extensive range, is maintained by hallucinations of sensation." He adds, "those who hear voices do not stop talking to their imagined conversational partners."[11] It is noteworthy that the physician seems to be a believer in Pinel's *moral treatment* as he quietly tries to correct the delusions of his patients, "the doctor goes from one to another, asking them questions [...] without forgetting to make tactful objections to each one."[12] Though, no doubt, aware of the chronicity and incurability of Rufete's delusions, he nevertheless attempts briefly to talk him out of them, "calm it, softly. If you could drop your [political] power for a few months how great it would be for both of us! We could concentrate on curing that upset completely."[13] The futility of his attempt is underlined by Rufete's immediate contradiction of his advice, and after signalling "there's no hope" to his companion, the physician goes on to the next patient.

Galdós's next verbal debt is to Esquirol as he describes the inhumane condition in which the non-paying poor, *pobres*, are housed at the hospital and, as narrator, reflects that even the sanest, on waking in such a

11 "Monomanías sensoriales ó alucinatorias-cuando el delirio de las ideas, sin ser difuso, sino manteniéndose circunscrito en una órbita más ó menos extensa, está sostenido por sensaciones alucinatorias" (*freno-patología* 449), "Los que oyen voces no cesan de hablar con sus fantásticos interlocutores" (*freno-patología* 450).

12 "El medico va de uno a otro, interrogándolos [...] sin dejar de hacer objeciones discretas a cada uno" (*desheredada* 69).

13 "Calma, serenedad. Si pudiera usted dejar el poder por unos cuantos meses, ¡qué bien nos vendría a los dos! Nos dedicaríamos a curar radicalmente ese constipado" (*desheredada* 70).

hen coop would, "surely become demented with the *monomanía* of being savage beasts."[14]

Up to this point, moral treatment and sedation have been employed without effect and Rufete becomes silent, withdrawn and emaciated, leading to a third variety of treatment, the high-pressure, cold-water shower. In this, the *médico* appears to be following established practice since Giné y Partagas observes, "As a method of control, the cold shower is one of the most powerful means, by which one can almost always overcome refusal to eat and obstinate refusal to talk ..." adding darkly, "Frequently it is enough to show the [the patient] the shower in order to get these results, and, at times, even the simple threat is enough."[15] Giné y Partagas summarizes his regime for the treatment of hallucinating mania, emphasizing the importance of hospital isolation, moral treatment (which he admits makes things worse in other hands), and intimidation of the patient with cold showers if he refuses to relinquish his delusional ideas. He adds that sedatives such as bromide may be useful for agitation and insomnia (460). From what he saw at Leganés, or from what he read, Galdós seems to be following Gine y Partagas' regime for Rufete to the letter.

Galdós's awareness of contemporary medical thinking is revealed even further as he describes the predisposing causes behind Rufete's mental derangement. Through his daughter Isidora's recollections of him, we learn that Rufete was secretary to three provincial governors and, according to her, would have been a governor himself had he not fallen foul of party politics (83). We are told that he was ambitious and was never content with his lot (82), that he felt that he would go mad if he did not achieve what he felt due to him (83), and that he was overwhelmingly obsessed with achieving the appearance of a notable person (83). Further details of mental instability in the Rufete's family emerge. One is revealed by Isidora's

14 "volviera seguramente a caer en demencia, con la monomanía de ser bestia dañina" (*desheredada* 71).

15 "Como medio de represión, el chorro frio es uno de los agentes más poderosos, con los cuales casi siempre se logra vencer la repulsión a tomar alimentos y el obstinado mutismo ... [...] Frecuentemente basta hacer presenciar el chorro, para lograr estos resultados, y aun á veces es suficiente la simple amenaza" (*freno-patología* 287).

seemingly incidental question to Canencia, the asylum bookkeeper, about Rufete's father, "His father, my grandfather, was also an official. The poor man died badly. Did you know him?[16] Galdós thus subtly informs us that Tomás' father had also been a patient at the asylum of Leganés and that he, too, had died there, implying a hereditary pattern of mental disturbance.[17] As the novel proceeds, Isidora's detachment from reality and her deeply rooted obsession with titled parentage are shown to be delusions that psychologically destroy her. These delusions appear as part of a pattern of degenerative, neurological dysfunction that extends thoughout the Rufete clan. Isidora's retarded brother Mariano, *Pecado*, is intellectually and emotionally retarded, is drawn irresistibly to the criminal underworld and, after escaping a capital sentence for the murder of a peer by reason of his young age, he finally meets his destiny with the garrotte as a failed regicide. Isidora's son, *Riquín*, is born with an abnormally large head (macrocephaly), seen at the time as an expression of degenerative, morbid heredity.[18] All these features appear in the medical literature of Galdós's time, and afford a narrative that accounts for Rufete's insanity.

16 "Su padre, mi abuelo, había sido también de oficina. El pobre murió de mala manera. ¿Le conoció usted?" (*desheredada* 83).

17 That such an implication was in Galdós's mind is revealed by Schnepf's study of the earlier manuscript version of *La desheredada* where Encarnación refers to Isidora's lineage, "your father, like your grandfather, like all the Rufetes ... a cursed breed of crazies," "tu padre, como tu abuelo, como todos los Rufetes ... maldita ralea de chiflados" (58). Ribbans comments in the context of the Captain Rufete who appears in Galdós's *Un faccioso más y algunos frailes menos* that, "[he] is not Tomás Rufete himself but his father. The link is significant, for it establishes a chain of deranged behaviour over three generations ..." (*History* 162).

18 Morel argues for progressive degeneration across the generations resulting in extinction through eventual sterility (*dégénérescence*, 683), and quotes abnormalities of the skull as a feature of this process (*maladies*, 585). Morel's work was extensively quoted by Galdós's contemporaries, Maudsley and Foville amongst them. Augusto Miquis appears to be aware of this hereditary progression, for he describes having told Isidora, half humorously perhaps, "your wild ambition and your psychological vice will give you a brood of weakly big-headed children ...," "su delirante ambición y su vicio mental le darán una descendencia de cabezudos raquíticos ..." (*desheredada* 290).

Many physicians of the day commented on the apparent increase in insanity in society. Morel in France observed an increase in mental disease associated with physical and moral ills (*Dégénérescences* vii), while Maudsley in England saw increasing numbers that he was unable to attribute simply to increased facilities for recognition and care (*Physiology* 202). In Spain, Hauser came to a similar conclusion (*siglo*, 202). The cause of this increase was frequently ascribed to the increasing complexity of nineteenth-century city life, with what Maudsley describes in Darwinian terms as, "a fierce and active struggle for existence" in which, "the weakest must suffer, and some of them break down into madness" (*Physiology* 202). Giné y Partagas denies that "civilization" in its best sense is related to mental disease, though implicitly admits that drunkenness, gambling and prostitution seen in the great cities were related to it (*frenopatología* 218–19). Closest to the vision of *La desheredada* is that of Hauser who saw in Spanish society "the excessive love of power and reputation, an unrestrained desire for [positions of] distinction and dignity, the unquenchable thirst for wealth and the love of luxury and pleasure; in a word ambition [...] giving rise to nervous stimulation that degenerates into mental disturbance."[19]

Among the causes of insanity, one that medical authorities agreed upon was heredity, and it was widely accepted that heredity was responsible for various anomalies affecting the nervous system. Giné y Partagas comments, "the morbid traits transmissible by heredity are varied; but in none [of them] is the influence of heredity so common as in mental disease."[20] Associated with this view was the idea that a familial nervous diathesis might be manifest as different psychiatric and neurological diseases in succeeding generations. Morel expanded his idea of degeneration in 1857

19 "el amor excesivo al poder y á la reputación, el deseo inmoderado de distinciones y dignidades, la sed insaciable de riquezas y el amor al lujo y al placer; en una palabra la ambición [...] dando lugar á excitaciones nerviosas que degeneran en aberraciones mentales" (*siglo* 339–40). Falret made identical observations on the causes of madness in French society 20 years earlier (xlvi).

20 "Varias son las aptitudes morbosas transmisibles por herencia; pero en ninguna el influjo hereditario en tan común como en la enajenación mental" (*freno-patología* 221).

and 1860, to include a large range of diseases that he thought transmissible by heredity, after having been acquired by antecedents as a result of physically or morally corrupting lives. Defining degenerates as those suffering from, "a pathological deviation from the normal type of humanity"[21] he expounds on the range of hereditable ills:

> It is not necessary [...] that the illness of the parents be *identically reproduced* in the children: *it suffices that the latter be endowed with an unfortunate organic predisposition that becomes the point of departure for pathological changes where the linkage and reciprocal effect produce new pathological states, be they physical, moral, and sometimes by a combination of both.*[22]

This idea was echoed later in Spain by Giné y Partagas, "the hereditary influence that predisposes to mental disease is not always manifest in ancestors by insanity since in many cases the disease of the latter is a neurological disease of a different order such as epilepsy, hysteria, chorea, etc."[23] Other contemporaries voiced similar opinions (Maudsley, *Physiology* 213, Foville 217, Guislain 431–33, Linas 162, Cotard 300), though with variations in the types of mental disturbance that they anticipated might appear in succeeding generations. In Foville's view, "certain illnesses, and especially

21 "una deviation maladive du type normal de l'humanité" (74). Morel attended seminary as a young man and would have been a priest had he not offended his superiors by his political views. He remained a deeply religious man, however, with a literal belief in *Genesis* such that, for him, the, "type normal de l'humanité" was that of man's primitive perfection from which degeneration represented a fall (Dowbiggin 118).

22 "Il n'est pas nécessaire [...] que la maladie des parents soit *identiquement reproduite* chez les enfants: *il suffit que ces derniers soit doués d'une prédisposition organique malheureuse que devienne le point de depart de transformations pathologiques dont l'enchaînement et la dépendance réciproque produisent de nouvelles entités maladives, soit de l'ordre physique, soit de l'ordre moral, et parfois des deux orders réunis*" (*Dégénérescences* 565, author's italics).

23 "no siempre el influjo hereditario que predispone á la enajenación mental se señala en los ascendentes por una vesania, sino que en muchos casos, la afección de estos consiste en una neuropatía de distinto orden, tal como la epilepsia, el histerismo, la corea, etc" (*freno-patología*, 222).

nervous diseases, can be transmitted from one generation to another, without remaining exactly the same in character,"[24] listing neurosis, epilepsy, hysteria, chorea and madness as examples. This narrative of morbid heredity permeates the story of *La desheredada*.

In Morel's view, poor diet, alcoholism, immorality, and unhealthy living and working conditions could be responsible for a pathological lineage, as he relied upon the widely held belief of his time in the inheritance of acquired characteristics. Morel explains, "it is not always necessary for them to reach the last degree of degradation for them to remain afflicted with sterility, and consequently incapable of transmitting their type of degeneration."[25] This is echoed by Maudsley in his "Ways of Avoiding Madness" that appeared in the *Revista Europa* in 1875. Maudsley sees hereditary transmission of degenerative mental disease as incontestable, "pathological evolution of the spirit across the generations, better expressed as pathological degeneration, is verifiably proven."[26] The idea was expressed in Spain in 1881 by Esquerdo as he analyses the insanity of the serial murderer-rapist Garayo, "the distinguished Morel affirms [...] that the descendants of chronic alcoholic parents [...] are frequently afflicted with the features of progressive degeneration."[27] Morelian doctrine forms the basis of the 1884 doctoral dissertation of the physician, Ramón Gómez Ferrer. It appears that Galdós also subscribes to the theory since in his report of the trial in 1886 of Cayetano Galeote, the assassin of the bishop of Madrid, he writes, "After hearing doctors Simarro and Vera, there is no doubt that Galeote is a

24 "certaines maladies, et spécialement les maladies nerveuses, peuvent se transmettre d'une generation à une autre, sans conserver exactement les mêmes caracteres" (218).

25 "il n'est pas toujours nécessaire qu'ils arrivent au dernier degré de la dégradation pour qu'ils restent frappés de stérilité, et consèquemment incapables de transmettre le type de leur dégénérescence" (*Dégénérescences* 5).

26 "Está probado que se verifica, a través de las generaciones, una evolución patológica del espíritu; ó mejor dicho, una degeneración patológica" (*medios* 411).

27 "El insigne Morel afirma [...] que los descendientes de padres entregados al alcoholismo crónico [...] ofrecen a menudo los caracteres de una degeneración progresiva" (*Locos* 25).

degenerate. His dementia is hereditary, many in his family having suffered overt insanity or other illnesses related to a diseased brain."[28]

Another development in European psychiatry in the nineteenth century was the recognition of patients who might perform violent crimes, such as murder, and yet appear to be otherwise rational. Pinel described this phenomenon as, *manie sans délire*,[29] Esquirol proposed a differently conceived entity of *monomanie-homicide*,[30] and James Cowles Prichard (1786–1848), acknowledging his debt to both *aliénistes*, referred to it as *moral insanity*.[31] While the entity was increasingly accepted in England and France, its use as a defence in the courts in Spain was opposed by traditional legal doctrine, much influenced by the Church, which held that unless the defendant was actually raving, he had to be considered to be responsible for his actions. In an attempt to reform this attitude, Esquerdo, Galdós's friend and Tolosa Latour's mentor, led a long and unsuccessful campaign to have criminal insanity recognized by the judiciary with the slogan of, "madmen who do not seem mad," *locos que no lo parecen*. Both Esquerdo and his former students acted as expert witnesses for the defence in a number of high-profile murder trials, though with little success in having their defendants referred to an asylum rather than to the garrotte.[32]

28 "No queda duda, después de oír a los doctores Simarro y Vera, que Galeote es un ser degenerado. Su demencia es hereditaria, y muchos individuos de esta familia han padecido locura manifiesta o bien otras enfermedades que tienen relación con los desórdenes encefálicos" (*Galeote* 179).

29 Pinel 155–60.

30 Goldstein observes that Esquirol departs from Pinel's concept of impulsive behaviour without any impairment of understanding, and claims that there was always some form of premonitory delirium (173).

31 Prichard 16.

32 The trials included those of the would-be regicide Otero, 1880 ("Causa de regicidio."), the serial murderer-rapist Garayo "Sacamantecas," 1881 (Becerro de Bengoa, "El Sacamantecas."), and the priest-assassin of the bishop of Madrid, Galeote 1886 (Pérez Galdós. "El crimen del cura Galeote"). Galdós thus not only reported on the trial of Galeote but, as Gordon shows, used Otero as the model of the would-be regicide, Mariano, in *La desheredada*. The course of Esquerdo's career as a defence witness is reviewed by Conseglieri and Villasante.

The portrayal of Mariano in *La desheredada*, with its parallels with the regicide Otero, appears to be influenced by the idea of moral insanity. At no point does Mariano suffer from psychosis or mania, but his emotional and intellectual retardation, associated with his epilepsy, argue for diminished responsibility. Galdós appears to argue for the inappropriateness of his execution, as Esquerdo pled for Otero and Garayo, and his disciples later claimed in their defence of Galeote.

Appearing three years after *La desheredada*, a different manifestation of psychological derangement, though also associated with inherited predisposition, occurs in *Lo prohibido*. In this novel, Galdós portrays the rational but disturbed character of José María Bueno de Guzmán, its central narrator and autobiographer. Set in Madrid in 1884, the novel is full of depictions of eccentricity, obsession and madness, where José María and his relations exhibit one or more of the three. From the beginning, José María confesses to subjective troubles that mark him as typical of his family. He suffers from attacks of hypochondria and nervous disorders, such as absence of appetite and insomnia, together with inexplicable attacks of anguished terror, more emotional than physical.[33] He complains of episodes of depression when he is overtaken by immense, irrational fear such as might be provoked by being in the path of an oncoming train. He finds himself so irritated by the sight of unfamiliar people that he has to fight to prevent himself from hitting them. This aggressive impulse even extends to his uncle Rafael who, in the face of such an unwelcoming reception, insists on visiting him. However, the visits are not intended to divert him with extraneous matters so much as to dwell on his symptoms, as if by so doing he might diminish them (136). Rafael quotes Augusto Miquis, whose fame as a physician is revealed later, as he labels José María as suffering from,

33 "más moral que física" (*prohibido* 135). In the nineteenth century the work *moral* also had the sense of emotional as well as moral in the ethical sense. The *moral treatment* of Pinel corresponds roughly to what would now be called psychotherapy (see Goldstein 80 ff.).

"the disease of the century that, by compelling mental activity, was creating a predisposition toward nervous disease in the entire human race."[34]

In his role as Job's comforter, Rafael regales José María with details of their psychiatrically flawed family in which disease traits are transmitted across the generations, in the same way that skin diseases and tuberculosis were considered to be inherited (136). The saga includes a wide range of extraordinary anomalies, ranging from a distant relative who wore a bedsheet in the streets at night to frighten the neighbours, to José María's own father who was a compulsive womanizer. A brother of Rafael developed a religious mania, later escaping from a religious seminary to marry a country girl, only to suffer later from severe anxiety. Another brother suffered depression to the extent that he ended up in an asylum, while a sister seemed to be normal, though had a phobia for dogs. She, in turn, produced a son who spent his life writing letters to himself.[35] The last surviving brother, Serafín, retired from a distinguished career as a naval officer only to develop compulsive kleptomania. We later discover that Serafín also has a penchant for chasing young women in the streets. Uncle Rafael claims that his own preoccupation with business has kept him on an even keel, but admits that he also suffers from attacks of anxiety as a result of excessive work. In these spells, his body feels suspended, a feeling lasting for several days.[36] Rafael completes the catalogue of living relatives with a sketch of his son, Raimundo, who is highly imaginative to the point of being dysfunctional, and who has aged prematurely. He describes his eldest daughter, María Juana, who is obsessed with a sensation of cloth in her mouth, and a middle daughter, Eloisa, with a phobia for feathers and flying creatures, and a constant feeling of a feather lodged in the throat. He concludes with

34 "el mal del siglo, el cual, forzando la actividad cerebral, creaba una diátesis neuropática constitutiva en toda la humanidad" (*prohibido* 136).

35 This character, Jesús Delgado, appears in *El doctor Centeno*.

36 Whiston notes that a patient described in Galdós's annotated copy of Armangué y Tuset suffered just such a sense of suspension in association with ophthalmic migraine (*Estudios* 141 n. 21). A sense of being suspended in space also appears in the description of *tabes dorsalis* in volume I of Jaccoud's *Tratado de patologia interna* (621), a text in Galdós's library.

his youngest daughter, Camila, who is so erratic in behaviour that an end in an asylum was feared for her, since she had been on the verge of suicide when her plans for marriage were frustrated.

Rafael reveals his dissatisfaction with the husbands of his three daughters and expresses an extraordinary flight of wishful thinking in which all his daughters might be rolled into one person who would then be able to marry José María. The latter finds this expression of Rafael's admiration for him so strange that he humorously recommends it to the attention of doctors who are involved in consultation on a case of neurosis. While he finds himself rejoicing at not being intimately involved with this family circle, José María finds Rafael's tale of family pathology so diverting that it produces in him a feeling of complete well-being.

Detailed consideration of José María's symptoms, suggests that his psychiatric disease is portrayed in the light of a recently described entity, *neurasthenia*, which enjoyed a vogue that endured for at least the following three decades.[37] The nosological concept was defined independently in 1869 by George Beard (1839–83) and Edwin Van Deusen (1828–1909) in the United States, and became particularly influential in Europe following its acceptance by Wilhelm Heinrich Erb (1840–1921) in Germany and its elaboration by Charcot in France in the later 1880s.[38]

Writing in the year that *Lo prohibido* was published, Hauser voices the widespread concern of his day about the increase in nervous diseases over the course of the previous half century. He describes the ubiquitous

37 Comenge uses the term in 1914 to describe a new type of patient, worn down by city life, being seen by doctors, "rebellious, neurasthenic, worn down by constant psycho-physical exhaustion," "insubordinado, neurasténico, agotado por el esquilmo psico-físico constante" (viii).

38 The European reception of neurasthenia is outlined by Marijke Gijswijt-Hofstra and Roy Porter. Beard wrote about well-to-do urban patients on the East Coast of the United States while Van Deusen described the condition in the rural poor of Michigan. The populations claimed to be at risk from this condition reflected these different patient groups. Beard claimed that neurasthenia ran a basically benign course in over-achieving professionals, while Van Deusen thought it frequently the prelude to frank insanity in the rural poor. Beard's place in nineteenth-century psychiatry is reviewed by Rosenberg (*Beard*).

complaint of "the nerves," and a striking increase in mental disease in the most recent 20 years (*siglo* 202–04). He comments further on the ambition, mental labour and nervous excitement experienced in contemporary urban life and the exhaustion that follows. These he links with:

> another disease, daughter of the nineteenth century, that is spreading increasingly every day in Europe and has been known for some time in the United States of America by the name of *Neurasthenia*, or weakness of the nervous system, an illness that, despite being very common among the inhabitants of large population centres, has hardly been described with the care it deserves in general texts of medicine. The American doctors Weir Mitchell and Beard are the only ones who have found it worthy of extensive monographs, while European medical specialists have always confused it, some with hysteria or with chloraemia, others with cerebral anaemia, yet others with spinal irritation.[39]

Hauser lists as predisposing causes of this exhaustion of nervous energy: sexual excess, multiple pregnancies, severe reverses of fortune and intellectual labour undertaken in childhood, outstripping physical resources

39 "otra enfermedad, hija del siglo XIX, que se extiende cada día más en Europa y hace tiempo es muy conocida en los Estados-Unidos de América con el nombre de *Neurastenia*, ó debilidad del sistema nervioso, enfermedad que, á pesar de ser muy común entre los habitantes de los grandes centros de población, apenas es descrita con el detenimiento que merece en las obras generales de Medicina. Los Doctores americanos Weir Mitchell y Beard son los únicos que la han encontrado digna de extensas monografías, mientras que los médicos especialistas europeos la han confundido siempre, unos con la histeria ó con la cloro-anemia, otros ya con la anemia cerebral, y con la irritación espinal" (*siglo* 206, author's italics). Hauser's confusion of the many subjective and poorly defined symptoms of neurasthenia with the supposedly organic "spinal irritation" may be forgiven since Beard himself repeatedly mentions the latter. Neurasthenia has since been described as giving patients a sense of suffering from physical disease, in contrast with similar symptoms of the hysteric, who was viewed as suffering from a poorly regarded, psychological process. A French neurological text by Grasset, available in Spanish translation in 1880, refers to neurasthenia as the "forma neurasthénica" of spinal cord disease, "in which the features of depression predominate rather than spinal irritation," "en que dominan los fenómenos de depression en lugar de irritación espinal" (vol 2, 208).

(*siglo* 206–07).[40] He stresses the great variety of symptoms, often seen in a combination unique to any given patient, which leads to prostration and complete inability to honour obligations. The visiting French-American psychiatrist Seguin found a perception among Spanish *alienistas* at the time that, "excessive intellectual exertion, caused by the greater competition of modern life" was responsible for the increased frequency of certain types of insanity. Ginè y Partagas informed Seguin that, "the anxiety and mental strain attending the increasingly severe struggle for existence is the chief cause" (412).

It is just such a nexus of civilization and progress that Beard in 1869 identifies as responsible for a wide range of subjective complaints such as dyspepsia, headache, insomnia, anaesthesia, neuralgia, hypochondriasis, loss of appetite, terrors, and roaring in the ears, that he bundles into the nosological entity of neurasthenia. He finds it, "most frequently met with in civilized, intellectual communities. They are part of the compensation for our progress and refinement" (*Neurasthenia* 217). He claims furthermore that "Neurasthenia may result from any causes that exhaust the nervous system. Hereditary descent terribly predisposes to neurasthenia, just as it predisposes to all forms of nervous derangement" (218). Without acknowledging his debt to Morel, he thus reveals his awareness of degeneration theory and polymorphous heredity by maintaining that, "sick headache, epilepsy or insanity or dyspepsia in the grandfather may skip over a generation and show itself as neurasthenia in the grandchildren" (218). He lists as additional causes, "pressures of bereavement, business and family cares, [...] sexual excesses, [...] and sudden retirement from business" (218), and summarizes it all, "the prime cause of modern nervousness is modern civilization with its accompaniments" (*Treatise* xv). Elsewhere he adds as

40 The Second Law of Thermodynamics, propounded by William Thompson, Lord Kelvin in 1862, explained entropy as an irreversible dissipation of energy in the universe. This concept was applied to medicine, where human energy was considered to be stored in finite and limited quantities. Henry Maudsley in 1874 referred to, "The energy of a human body being a definite and not inexhaustible quantity," and he questions whether the young can, "bear, without injury, an excessive mental drain as well as the natural physical drain which is so great at that time" (*Sex*, 199).

predisposing influences, "steam power, the periodical press, the telegraph, the sciences, and the mental activity of women" (*American* vi). Neurasthenia can, then, be well summarized as "a disorder of modernity, caused by the fast pace of urban life."[41]

The relief provided to José María by Rafael's relation of family illnesses is not long-lasting, for after various business trips, his symptoms recur. He returns to Madrid with a low grade fever that his doctor, Moreno Rubio, finds reminiscent of malaria, *paludismo*. The fever is resistant to the anti-malarial drug, *la quinina*, and was apparently acquired in the Pyrenees, an area usually not notable for its marshes or malaria (*prohibido* 179).[42] The illness goes on for weeks with periods of improvement and recurrence that Moreno treats by advising rest and patience. These were the mainstays of the treatment of neurasthenia.

José María repeats the catalogue of features of his "lamentable nervous state," "the villainous chronic nervous indisposition that appeared with its thoroughbred symptoms."[43] He lists inexplicable, unfocused terror, which his doctor attributes not to failing of his reason (with its implication of incipient insanity), but to unbalanced nutrition. This is of little consolation to José María, however, who also complains of lack of appetite. He goes on to detail dizziness, insomnia and irritability together with ceaseless, varied noises in the ears that keep him awake at night. We learned earlier that cousin Raimundo is given to reading medical texts (*prohibido* 170) so might recognize from his researches a possible diagnosis of José María's complaints. Raimundo describes, "a manifestation of the listless state, a pathological feature of large urban populations of the nineteenth century.

41 Gijswijt-Hofstra 1.

42 This isolated reference to malaria in *Lo prohibido* is of interest in that malaria-like symptoms in neurasthenia are mentioned by both Beard (*treatise* 59, 69) and Van Deusen (5), a suggestion of the detail of Galdós's research.

43 "la picara desazón crónica, que apareció con sus síntomas castizos" (179). Galdós may be indulging in a play on words here as *castizo* may indicate "pure" to suggest "typical symptoms," with an additional sense of symptoms of the well-born. Beard was at pains to emphasize the superior social and intellectual qualities of his neurasthenic patients, an association which they found agreeable.

Little, feverish energy to start off with, little, healing energy afterwards, with debility all the time."[44] It sounds very much as if Raimundo has been reading a text by Beard. When we add three other features that Beard lists, bereavement, terrible noises in the ears and retirement from business, the impression is strengthened further that Galdós was influenced by contemporary descriptions of neurasthenia.

By the end of the novel, José María's obsessional affairs with his two older married cousins and his wilful inability to comprehend Camila's integrity, and her refusal to be seduced by him, cause him to suffer a stroke. In a state of terminal exhaustion, he completes his memoir, which is to be published posthumously. Galdós will not let his depiction of the stroke pass, with its mention of transient paralysis of the left side of the body (hemiparesis) without subtle features that further reveal the unusual extent of his research.

As José María gradually recovers from his hemiparesis and struggles to regain his faculties, he records an unusual experience. When visited by his cousins María-Juana, Eloísa and Camila, all of whom he has very good reason to know well, he finds that he cannot recognize their faces:

> But on the second night, the saddest example of this loss of faculties was not to recognize those three women who I saw in a row in front of me. As I awoke from one of those lethargic spells, they came to my attention and I said to myself, "I know these faces; I have seen them somewhere" [...] those three faces and upper bodies were not unfamiliar to me; but my brains burned in a furious effort of enquiry, without being able to clarify who they were or what their names were.[45]

44 "una manifestación del estado adinámico, carácter patológico del siglo XIX en las grandes poblaciones. Poca fuerza febril primero, poca fuerza reparatriz después, debilidad siempre" (*prohibido* 179).

45 "Pero el ejemplo más triste de esta pérdida de la facultad fue no saber quiénes eran aquellas tres mujeres a quienes vi la segunda noche, en fila delante de mí. Ofreciéronse a mi atención al despertar de uno de aquellos letargos, y me dije: 'Yo conozco estas caras; las he visto en alguna parte' [...] aquellas tres caras y aquellos tres bustos no me eran desconocidos; pero mi cerebro ardía en un trabajo furioso de indagación, sin poder sacar en claro quiénes eran ni cómo se llamaban" (591).

José María gradually recovers his powers of recognition, to the point where he can finally recognize the cousins who have played such a dominant part in his recent life.

Remarkably, what Galdós is describing here is the syndrome of inability to recognize faces, or *prosopagnosia* (Greek *prosop*=face, person, *agnosia*=unknown). While the condition is more commonly congenital, it can rarely be seen as a complication of stroke and follows damage to the right side of the brain, which may result in left hemiparesis, as Galdós describes in José María.[46] As Galdós expresses it through José María, a sense of familiarity may exist without actual recognition of the faces of people otherwise very well known to him.[47] While the term *prosopagnosia* was coined by Bodamer as recently as 1947,[48] the condition was described at least as early as 1844 by Wigan.[49] It was also the subject of case reports of inability to recognize a more extensive range familiar objects by the English neurologist, John Hughlings Jackson (1835–1911), in 1876 and by Charcot in France in 1883. While it is possible that the half-French Tolosa Latour knew of Charcot's description, if not those in the English literature,[50] it is, perhaps, more likely that Galdós may have learned about of this rare condition as a result of being shown a patient, or being told about it, by his medical friends.

46 The well-known neurologist and author, Oliver Sacks, suffers from congenital prosopagnosia and has written about his experience of the condition.

47 "The two have different neural bases and can be dissociated; thus, although both are lost in tandem with prosopagnosia, one can have familiarity without recognition or recognition without familiarity in other conditions" (Sacks 41).

48 Bodamer, J. "Die Prosop-Agnosie." *Archiv für Psyhiatrie und Nervenkrankenheit* 179 (1947): 6–54. A translation and review in English were published by Ellis and Florence in 1990.

49 "A gentleman of middle age […] lamented to me his utter inability to remember faces […] and it was not until he heard the voice, that he could recognize men with whom he had constant intercourse" (170).

50 The descriptions of loss of face-recognition of Charcot and Hughlings Jackson are repeatedly quoted in the literature on prosopagnosia, but both record it in association with loss of recognition of other visual stimuli such as colours and non-human objects. Neither account is as specific to the face as that of Wigan's patient.

An entirely different depiction of insanity is to be found in one of Galdós's most detailed clinical portraits, that of Maximiliano Rubín in *Fortunata y Jacinta*, whose underlying physical condition is analysed in Chapter 3. We know from what Galdós tells us of Maxi's family, from the story of his youth and his physical appearance that he is depicted as suffering from the delayed, congenital form of syphilis, the condition first recognized by Jonathan Hutchinson nearly 30 years before *Fortunata* was composed. This form of congenital syphilis, affecting tissues throughout the body as it does, is equivalent to the tertiary forms of the adult-acquired disease.

Galdós's describes a deteriorating psychosis that has many of the features of G.P.I. He portrays Maxi as emotionally unstable and prepared to contemplate both murder and suicide, for he says to Fortunata, "Ah! A revolver … – Yes to kill you and me."[51] He experiences spells of depressive withdrawal at some times, and manic excitement at others. In addition, he endures episodes of paranoia, being convinced at one moment that his family intends to poison him, "this chocolate contains arsenic."[52] On another occasion he is consumed with a passion for logical analysis, "he was overcome by a mania for logic,"[53] while at other times he has delusions of religious grandeur, "I am no more than the forerunner of this doctrine; the doctrine's true Messiah will come later, will come soon; is already on the way. He who knows all has told me."[54] He has a hallucination of an insubstantial presence in his bedroom, "the day before yesterday in this very bedroom there was the impression, yes, the impression of a person […] it was like imprints left in the air, like a smell, like the shape of a body in the atmosphere."[55] In complete contrast with this, he is later able to describe

51 "¡Ay!, un revólver … – Sí, para matarte y matarme" (*Fortunata I* 703).

52 "Este chocolate tiene arsénico" (*Fortunata II* 279).

53 "le sobrevino el *furor de la lógica*" (*Fortunata II* 417, author's italics).

54 "Yo no soy más que el precursor de esta doctrina; el verdadero Mesías de ella vendrá después, vendrá pronto; ya está en camino. Quien todo se lo sabe me lo ha dicho a mí" (*Fortunata II* 307).

55 "Y anteayer había en esa misma alcoba la impresión, sí, la impresión de una persona […] era como huellas dejadas en el aire, como un olor, como el molde de un cuerpo en el ambiente" (*Fortunata II* 277).

his experience of his disturbed mental states in a lucid interval that has all the appearance of rationality, "First I suffered a delirium of persecution, then of grandeur … I invented religions […] I suffered homicidal mania, and nearly killed my aunt and *Papitos*. Terrible depression followed by yearning to die, a religious mania […] and deliria of abnegation and release …"[56]

A very full description of the psychiatric features seen in G.P.I., is given by Giné y Partagas: paranoia, hallucinations, megalomania, religious delusions, mania, depression, violence and a remittent course with temporary lucid intervals that may give an (illusory) hope of a cure (*freno-patología* 529–46). Such a list suggests how comprehensively Galdós portrayed Maxi, based upon features of the disease recognized in his time. In addition, obsessively logical reasoning was listed in 1880 by Vera, who also mentions diffuse interstitial periencephalitis, diffuse interstitial encephalitis and softening of the brain, *reblandecimiento*, as features of G.P.I., *parálisis general* (56, 75, 78, 60). The cerebral softening that Ballester, Maxi's mentor in the pharmacy, suggests as a possible diagnosis, is also listed as a feature of G.P.I. in the writings of Giné y Partagas (*freno-patología* 539) and Fournier (*cerveau* 68–69). The condition was recognized as commonplace in hospitals of Galdós's time. Hauser estimated in 1884 that 20–25% of asylum patients in Europe suffered from it (*siglo* 205–06), and it must have been well-known to Galdós's medical friends and informants, especially to Vera. The detail of Galdós's description of Maxi's syphilis and his madness indicate the depth of his research into what was then a tragically common and incurable condition.[57]

In addition to his depiction of madness in major characters such as Maxi, Galdós was quite prepared to describe eccentricity verging on

56 "Primero tuve el delirio persecutorio, después el delirio de grandezas … Inventé religiones […] Padecí también furor de homicidio, y por poco mato a mi tía y a Papitos. Siguieron luego depresiones horribles, ganas de morirme, manía religiosa […] y el delirio de la abnegación y el desprendimiento …" (*Fortunata II* 491).

57 Given the likelihood that Galdós developed *tabes dorsalis* in his later years and the long latent period of the disease of up to 30 years after initial infection, it is not entirely unlikely that, while he was composing *Fortunata y Jacinta*, he had personal as well as novelistic motives for researching syphilis as thoroughly as he did.

madness in secondary characters. He does so most entertainingly in his portrait of doña Isabel Godoy in *El doctor Centeno*. Doña Isabel is the great aunt of Alejandro Miquis, Felipe Centeno's second master. She is prey to obsessive cleanliness and spends much of her time dusting and polishing her home with the aid of her maid, Teresa, "She had a fanaticism that dominated her, that of cleanliness [...] complete cleaning [of the house] was performed daily. Doña Isabel had a maidservant [...] and between them they shared the work equally."[58] Doña Isabel refuses to eat any food that is not prepared from ingredients brought to her from her former home town of Toboso, and cooked in the Manchegan style. In the matter of drink, she confines herself to various forms of herbal tea.

As a young woman she had grown up reading romantic novels that consumed her imagination, a clear novelistic homage to Don Quijote (256). Disappointed in love, she becomes convinced that she is the incarnation of her dead sister, "with her spirit endlessly saturated with the memory of her sister she achieved the psychological phenomenon of transubstantiation [...] and had come to say almost without thinking about it: 'I am Piedad ... I am my sister ...'"[59] In addition, she believes herself to be endowed with second sight by virtue of having been born on Holy Thursday, saying to her ill-fated great-nephew, "Beware, Alejandro ... do not behave badly ... remember that I was born on Holy Thursday and will be watching you constantly ..."[60] With a knowing wink both at the Quijote and at his own *La desheredada*, Galdós has Alejandro's father write to him with a report by a Tobosa neighbour (highly eccentric in his own right) about doña Isabel's mental health, "Don Santiago Quijano has told me that the poor

58 "Tenía un fanatismo que la avasallaba, el de la limpieza ... La limpieza general se hacía diariamente [...] Tenía doña Isabel una criada [...] y entre ambas se repartían el trabajo por igual" (*Centeno* 252).

59 "... empapando sin cesar su espíritu en la memoria de su hermana, había logrado realizar el fenómeno psicológico de la transubstanciación [...] había llegado a decir casi sin pensarlo: – 'Yo soy Piedad ... yo soy mi hermana ...'" (*Centeno* 258).

60 "¡Mira, Alejandro, que yo he nacido en Jueves Santo! ... Tú no seas malo ... Mira que te estoy mirando siempre" (*Centeno* 278).

thing is absolutely mad. Poor lady! Visit her and help her all you can and treat her with tact so as not to offend her."[61]

Thus far Galdós has regaled us with a highly entertaining portrait of extreme eccentricity extending to an inoffensive form of madness. What may relate this to the medical context of his time, however, is that doña Isabel's madness has communicated itself to her maid, Teresa:

> The maid, who had served [doña Isabel] for many years was a mature woman [...] Life shared with doña Isabel had caused her to assimilate with her to an astonishing degree. First of all she adopted the scruples, then the tastes, the habits, and finally the manner of speech and even the facial expression ... Finally they were like friends between whom everything was shared, work, food, prayer and even thoughts.[62]

The phenomenon of a previously sane person acquiring the delusions of a mad individual with whom they live in close personal contact has been recognized anecdotally for many years. In medical science, however, it appears under the the name of *folie à deux*, following its description by Lasègue and Falret in 1877 some six years before *El doctor Centeno* was published.[63] These authors summarize their impressions of the circumstances when *la contagion de la folie* takes place, finding it when two persons live in close contact for a prolonged period in which they share the same interests, feelings and beliefs (296). They describe the more intelligent, "active" person of the pair gradually imposing his or her delusions upon the weaker or

61 "Ha llegado D. Santiago Quijano y me ha dicho que la pobre está rematadamente loca. ¡Pobre señora! Visítala; sírvele en lo que puedas y trátala con tacto y estudio para no ofenderla" (*Centeno* 261–62).

62 "La criada, que desde luengos años la servía, era una mujer de bastante edad [...] La comunidad de vida con doña Isabel habíala asimilado pasmosamente con esta. Pegáronsele primero los escrúpulos, luego los gustos, las costumbres, y por último, el modo de hablar y hasta la fisonomía ... Últimamente, eran como amigas, y todo era en ellas común, el trabajo, la comida, los rezos y hasta los pensamientos" (*Centeno* 254).

63 In his review of *folie à deux* in 1880, Régis notes the contribution to knowledge of the condition in the context of paranoia, "dèlire de la persecution" by Legrand du Saulle in 1871. Régis stresses the identical nature of the delusion of the couple, "est constituée par un délire similaire, absolutment identique" (8).

"passive" person (296). A characteristic of the communicable delusions is that they must be more or less plausible.[64] Though seen in both sexes, the authors found the condition more common in women.

It would appear that news of the newly identified psychiatric entity spread quickly, since a reference to it, attributed to Lasègue and Legrande du Saule, appears in Spanish in Giné y Partagas' text a year before the Lasègue's article. In Giné's description of varieties of monomania, he confirms that the entity had long been recognized proverbially before its formal description in the medical literature:

> The influence of *imitation* has been observed on various occasions hence the proverbial saying *one madman makes a hundred*, which must relate to the tendency for monomania to be communicated emotionally. The *madness in pairs*, which Lasegue and Legrande du Saulle have described, is simply monomania that spreads to those who live in intimate contact with this type of insane patient.[65]

Galdós may well have had an opportunity to observe for himself the *folie à deux* upon which to base this wonderful picture of the Quixotically mad doña Isabel. The rapid spread of knowledge of the entity to Spain, and the very precise correspondence of fictional characters with the medical description, however, suggest that it may be another instance of Galdós's unrecognized awareness of contemporary medicine.

64 "c'est que ce délire ait un caractère de vraisemblance" (296).

65 "En diferentes ocasiones se ha observado el influjo de la *imitación*, y si por algo se ha dicho proverbialmente que *un loco hace ciento*, debe ser con relación á lo que puede el contagio moral de la monomanía. La *locura de dos*, que han descrito Lasegue y Legrande du Saulle, no es más que la monomanía que se propaga á las personas que viven en íntimo consorcio con locos de esta clase" (*freno-patología* 441, author's italics).

CHAPTER 6

Eye Disease and Blindness

Blindness is the most common physical disability to be portrayed in Galdós's novels, leading some to wonder if it might have been a premonitory preoccupation of the author.[1] Chamberlin, however, makes a convincing case to suggest that its frequency reflected the very high incidence of visual impairment among the mendicant poor on the streets of Madrid where Galdós set most of his novels.[2] The relatively high incidence of blindness in the Spanish capital was part of a national problem; Jimeno Agiús' study of the 1877 census finds a higher frequency of blindness in Spain than in any other European country.[3] In addition to its own indigent population, Madrid attracted beggars of all kinds from the provinces where resources were even more slender. Among these, nearly 30 per 10,000 inhabitants were blind.[4] Most of Galdós's characters with deteriorating vision or blindness appear in novels that were composed before the author's own visual problems became troublesome.

Chamberlin observes that in Galdós's novels, the characters' blindness frequently serves as a metaphor for inability to see beyond their mentally

1 "an undoubtedly premonitory character" "un indudable carácter premonitoria" (Barbón-Garcia *et al.* 551). Galdós suffered from deteriorating vision, which could not be corrected by spectacles, by the turn of the century. According to Herrera Hernández, the ophthalmologist Manuel Marquez diagnosed bilateral cataracts with inflammation of the iris (iritis) of the left eye in about 2006 (*Consideraciones* 23). In 1911 and 1912 cataract surgery on both eyes was unsuccessful; thereafter Galdós was blind.

2 See Chamberlin, particularly chapter 2.

3 *población* 362.

4 *población* 578–581. Of the 49 cities and regions listed by Jimeno only 3 (Almería, Alicante and Murcia) had greater proportions of the blind.

imposed confines: that of religious conservatism (Juan de Lantigua in *Gloria*) for example, or of social caste (Rafael de Águila in the *Torquemada* novels). Similarly, the blindness of the Conde de Albrit in *El abuelo* symbolizes inability to see beyond the traditional code of honour into the realities of the human heart.[5] On the other hand, Galdòs appears to mencion some blind characters, identified only as *ciegos*, to add authenticity to his descriptions of the streets of Madrid as he knew them.[6]

Galdós continues to reveal his knowledge of medicine in the context of other characters with ophthalmic disease, however. In *La desheredada*, Galdós endows Juan Bou, the Catalán lithographer-printer with nystagmus in his single functioning eye for he has, "two unequal eyes, one very lively with a slight rotatory movement, the other fixed and without lustre."[7]

This unusual ocular abnormality suggests a possible relation with the trial in Vitoria in 1880 of the notorious serial murderer and rapist Garayo, *el Sacamantecas*, which resulted in a capital sentence on 11th November executed in the following May. While the trial may have attracted limited attention in Madrid, Garayo became better known in the capital as a result of a series of well-publicised conferences given by Esquerdo, who had not only defended Garayo but continued his campaign to have criminal insanity recognized by the Spanish courts. He had given his "Madmen who don't seem Mad," *Locos que no lo parecen*, lecture in early 1880 following his unsuccessful defence of a would-be regicide Franciso Otero.[8] As a result of

5 I do not study the blindness in these major characters, nor that of Almudena in *Misericordia* or Lucía in *Ángel Guerra*, since Galdós portrays them with little detail of the medical conditions that gave rise to their loss of sight.

6 One might mention as examples the, "blind men tapping the ground with sticks, maimed […] horrible faces," "ciegos iban dando palos en el suelo, lisiados […] horribles caras" (*Fortunata I* 323), also "a blind girl asking for alms, 'una ciega que pedía limosna,'" who Moreno-Isla gives a pittance to, only to regret his meanness later (*Fortunata II* 361).

7 "dos ojos desiguales, el uno vivísimo, dotado de un ligero movimiento rotatorio, el otro fijo y sin brillo" (*desheredada* 322).

8 The trial was reported in *El Liberal* ("Causa de regicidio") on 7th February 1880, while Esquerdo's conference was summarized by Tejada y España in the following month (*Locos* 144–45).

what he maintained was a similar miscarriage of justice, Esquerdo repeated his Otero lecture, but with Garayo as its focus.[9]

The lecture was delivered in the first months of 1881 at the same time that Galdós was writing the second part of *La desheredada*. Esquerdo describes the hereditary and physical abnormalities of the accused, among which he includes his involuntary, repetitive and rotatory eye movements, "his gaze ... has a wild, wounding intensity and when he directs it laterally a symptom becomes more marked that in our medical jargon we call rotatory *nystagmus*, which is none other than a rotatory movement which accentuates increasingly the sinister nature of that gaze."[10]

The condition of nystagmus was well-recognized in medical circles at the time and was classified according to the plane of oscillation as horizontal, vertical or rotatory, although a mixed type of movement was occasionally recorded. It was seen in subjects with poor vision, in those with intracranial haemorrhage or infection, and in miners who spend their lives working in very dim light. It could also be seen early in life as an inherited form.[11] The latter was considered by some physicians to be a stigma of inherited degeneration, and Warlomont quotes Legrand du Saulle, an *aliéniste* who trained under Morel:

> Nystagmus is one of the stigmata of pathological inheritance. It is a *taint* that rarely occurs alone and is often found with many other physical signs (tics, facial asymmetry, cranial malformations, deformities of the ears etc., etc.). Clearly one cannot maintain that the individual with nystagmus is destined to go mad! One is simply saying that nystagmus is one of the signs of brain heredity and that this particular state is almost always found among those who have come from mentally disturbed families.[12]

9 The lecture was reported by Ángel Pulido in *El siglo médico* on 10 February 1881 (*Locos*), and by Tejada y España on 31 January 1881 (*Conferencia*).

10 "su mirada ... tiene una fiera intensidad que hiere, y cuando la dirige hácia los lados se acentúa más un síntoma que en nuestra jerigonza médica llamamos *nistagmus* rotatorio que no es otra cosa que un movimiento giratorio que acentúa más y más lo siniestro de aquella mirada" (*Locos* 15, author's italics).

11 Abadie 219–26.

12 "Le nystagmus est l'un des stigmates de l'hérédité pathologique. C'est une *tare* qui existe rarement isolée et que l'on retrouve réunie à beaucoup d'autres signes physiques

Such an opinion leads one directly to the major Galdós character with nystagmus, Leré in *Angel Guerra*. In the first description of her, the unusual behaviour of her eyes receives detailed attention for they are, "affected by a constitutional movement, an oscillation in the horizontal plane which resembles clockwork dolls which, impelled by their mechanism, move the pupils from right to left [...] which is scientifically known as *rotatory nystagmus*."[13] Galdós makes it clear that this condition is an example of the pathology that affects so many characters in the novel, for he gives her in addition a, "tic or habit of blinking incessantly"[14] that, in combination with her nystagmus, is enough to make people talking to her feel dizzy or even sick. This is exactly the combination of features that Legrand du Saulle thought was indicative of inherited cerebral abnormality. Galdós quotes the folk tradition of *maternal impression* to account for Leré's ocular abnormalities, "they say that the cause of the nervous affliction was that

---

(tics, asymétrie faciale, malformations crâniennes, deformation des oreilles etc., etc.). Évidament l'on ne saurait prétendre que l'individu qui est attaint de nystagmus est destine à perdre la raison! On dit simplement que le nystagmus est l'un des signes d'une hérédité cérébral, et que cet état particulier se rencontré presque toujours chez ceux qui sont issus de familles *incorrects* au point de vue mental" (835, author's italics). The author cites as his source Legrand du Saulle's *De la folie héréditaire* (1873), but I have been unable to identify the quotation in this text. The idea would have familiar to physicians of Galdós's day, however, and we can assume it to have been in circulation in Spain as it was in France. Deval lists, "other nervous diseases [...] insanity" as being associated with nystagmus (768), while in 1898 Féré continues to list nystagmus as one of the stigmata of familial degeneration (312).

13 "afectados de una movilidad constitutiva, de una oscilación en sentido horizontal, que la asemejaba á esos muñecos de reloj, que al compás del escape mueven las pupilas de derecha á izquierda [...] que científicamente se denomina *nistagmus rotatorio*" (76, author's italics). In the interests of strict accuracy, I have to point out that what Galdós is describing here is nystagmus that is *horizontal* not *rotatory*. Lucille Braun records an interview with Gregorio Marañón in 1957 when he recalled that the creation of Leré was influenced by a real-life original, "she was a Sta. de Lobo, from Avilés, who entered a convent some two years before the novel was written. She suffered from the same eye defect, *nistagmus rotatorius* (author's italics) that fascinated all who met Leré" (33 n.4).

14 "tic ó maña de pestañear incesantemente" (*Guerra* 76).

when her mother was pregnant, she suffered a great shock [with the result that] the child was born with that vibration of the optic nerves."[15] Galdós makes it clear when Leré recounts the history of her family that the cause, in the understanding of the time, was deeply rooted in her family history with its many hallmarks of inherited degeneration.

Leré's father was a severe alcoholic and the first four children born to her mother were "monsters" of whom only one, Juan, survives. Juan is severely disabled such that his lower body is wasted and soft as if it contains no bones, both arms like the legs resembling flaccid pillow slips. While his head is commensurate with his age of 25 years, his body is that of a child.[16] Leré is the fifth child and is followed by a brother, Sabas, *el nuevo Mozart*, who is such an extraordinary musical prodigy that he, too, is described as a monster for being so unusual.[17] Lere's abnormalities goes well beyond the ocular, however, as she also has visions of the Virgin Mary, by whom she

15 "Cuentan que la causa de tal afección nerviosa fué que, hallándose su madre embarazada, tuvo un gran susto y la criatura salió con aquella vibración de los nervios ópticos" (*Guerra* 76). The history of the ancient belief that a stressful experience endured by a pregnant mother can produce abnormalities in the unborn child is described by Bondeson.

16 Moreau de Tours quotes his colleague Morel, since both were convinced of the existence of trans-generational degeneration consequent upon alcohol abuse. Moreau writes, "If congenital imbecility and idiocy are extremes amongst the descendants of alcoholics, the observer will see a large number of intermediate states through aberrations of intelligence and through perversions," "Si l'imbécilité congénitale, l'idiotie, sont les termes extremes de la dégradation chez les descendants d'individus alcoolisés, un gran nombre d'états intermédiaires se révèlent à l'observateur par les aberrations de l'intelligence et par des perversions" (156).

17 Unusually gifted individuals were thought to come from families with a higher incidence of insanity and mental deficiency, since both deviations from the normal were thought to be related. Moreau de Tours published this theory in 1859, "it is amongst the classes of society that include men most distinguished for their outstanding talents of intelligence that one finds the most insane," "c'est parmi les classes de la société qui comptent le plus d'hommes distingués par les qualities éminents de leur intelligence que se trouvent le plus d'aliénés" (507). Magnan, a degenerationist of the following generation, felt constrained to create a category of "superior degeneration" to accommodate the genius. For a fuller discussion see Huertas (*Madness*).

has been advised to adopt a life of passive, abnegating asceticism. In addition to this existence devoid of pleasure or happiness, she believes that she should seek a slavery of pain, suffering and humiliation (139). Furthermore, she suffers a prolonged epileptic convulsion in her paroxysm of grief at the death of Ángel's daughter, Ción (175). Galdós thus shows us that Lere's nystagmus is but the most obvious sign of a deep-seated degenerative constitution, and that her masochistic religiosity is also likely to be pathological.[18]

In the very different universe of *Marianela* (1878) Galdós places the issue of blindness centre-stage as he portrays the disability of Pablo Penáguilas, a privileged young man, or *señorito*, of about 20. He is the only son of the widowed Francisco Penáguilas, who is lives comfortably on inherited money in the village of Aldeacorba not far from the iron mines of Socartes. Pablo is intelligent, inquisitive and exceptionally good looking (109),[19] but has been completely blind since birth as a result of congenital cataracts.[20] He walks about the surrounding countryside guided by an ugly, ignorant and poor girl of about sixteen, who is, however, sweet-hearted and completely devoted to him.[21] Pablo and Marianela spend much time is each other's company and declare strong affection for each other, to the extent that Pablo not only offers her education and a home and but also declares his love (125) and privately proposes marriage to her (133).

18 The OED records the first use of the word, "masochism" in 1890 in Krafft-Ebing's *Neue Forschungen auf dem Gebiet der Psychopathia Sexualis* at the time that *Ángel Guerra* was being written. It seems probable, however, that Galdós heard of, or encountered, this type of behaviour seen in Leré before the term was coined.

19 All pages of *Marianela* cited are those of the Cátedra text of 2003 edited by Francisco Caudet, hereafter *Marianela*.

20 Golfín later comments, "Our blind man is able to perceive no light at all," "Nuestro ciego no percibe claridad alguna" (*Marianela* 159) and comments that, "the visible world is absolutely unknown to him" (*Marianela* 153).

21 Even Marianela's champion, Teodoro Golfín, who recognizes her sensibility and imagination, "born to be good" understands that she is naïve, superstitious and deprived, "impaired by the savage state in which you have lived, by abandonment and absence of education, lacking the barest necessities," "desvirtuada por el estado salvaje en que has vivido, por el abandono y la falta de instrucción, pues careces hasta de la más elemental" (*Marianela* 213).

Into this rural idyll arrives Teodoro Golfín, brother of the mine manager, Carlos, who Galdós describes as having achieved the pinnacle of expertise as an ophthalmic surgeon as a result of great determination and wide professional experience acquired in travel abroad.[22] Golfín arrives with the intention of removing of Pablo's cataracts and giving him sight, which he learns will be a pre-condition for Pablo's family-arranged marriage to his rich and beautiful cousin, Florentina. The operation is a complete success with Pablo revelling in visual reality for the first time. He is immediately endowed with a sense of visual aesthetics that enables him to appreciate his cousin's good looks, as a result of which he declares his passionate devotion to her. In contrast, he is shocked to discover how ugly Marianela appears. Despite his attempts to disguise his obvious distaste for her, Marianela is deeply wounded and enters a decline from which none can save her. She finally expires as she symbolically joins the hands of the two beautiful lovers upon her chest.

So many elements enter into this sentimental story that it has led critics to categorize it in various ways. On the one hand, the vivid descriptions of the Socartes mines have a documentary Naturalistic quality about them that has elicited comparison with Zola's descriptions of the mine workings in *Germinal* (Caudet, *Introducción* 36). The utter misery of the mineworkers' life, represented by the Centeno dwelling where Marianela lives, is contrasted with the Penáguilas' comfortable bourgeois life, which is based on inherited wealth. The study of such embedded social injustice seems to belong to the *novela de tesis* genre exemplified by *Gloria* and *La*

22 Ophthalmology as a distinct specialty in Spain was still being consolidated at the time that Galdós wrote *Marianela* and training abroad was considered highly desirable, since, "in Spain the teaching [of ophthalmology] was characterized during the Restoration by inertia and absence of innovation," "En España, la enseñanza durante el período de la Restauración se caracteriza por la atonía y la falta de renovación" (Munoa and Cotallo 181). Munoa writes of, "the first generation of Spanish ophthalmologists, worthy of the name, were all doctors with an excellent scientific training in various European clinics, above all in Paris," "la primera generación de oftalmólogos españoles merecedores de tal título, son médicos poseedores, todos, de una excelente formación científica en diversas clínicas europeas, de preferencia en París" (55).

familia de Leon Roch, between which *Marianela* was written. Strong elements of romantic idealism and philosophical symbolism have been seen in the novel by some critics (Ruiz, Casalduero 204–21) and contested by others (Eoff 132–33, Jones).[23] While the novel begins with Naturalistic veracity, at other times the story takes on the quality of a romantic fable that cannot be taken literally, and it ends in melodrama as Marianela enters her final decline. Another critic relates the novel to Galdós's nostalgia for the idealized lost love of his cousin Sisita in early life.[24] With such dissension, it seems clear that no single category can adequately account for the novel and that many literary genres may be involved.

Given this rich but potentially confusing profusion of novelistic elements, it is, perhaps, unsurprising that Galdós's medical account of Pablo Penáguilas' blindness should be similarly mixed at literal and symbolic levels. Galdós had clearly studied the ophthalmology of his time and gives Teodoro Golfín a convincing vocabulary to explain the technical problem that he faced.[25] As the story proceeds, however, it veers into a non-literal and more symbolic account of medical matters. One suspects that Galdós knew it to be highly implausible, but that the literal had to be sacrificed for the integrity of his romantic story.

Having arrived at Aldeacorba to meet the Penáguilas family and reunite with his brother, Teodoro Golfín shares with the family the remarkable story of his rise from poverty to distinction in the field of ophthalmic surgery.[26]

23 After admitting the presence of symbolism in *Marianela*, Montesinos warns of the difficulty of their interpretation, "this [matter] of symbols is slippery ground," "esto de los símbolos es terreno escurridizo" (*I* 238).

24 "[*Marianela*] is Galdós's romantic novel, the compensation for frustrated, impossible love, supreme purity that was embodied in a fictional world thanks to this ideal figure," "ésta [*Marianela*] es la romántica de Galdós, la compensación por el amor frustrado; el imposible amor, la suprema pureza se incorporaron al orbe ficticio gracias a esta figura ideal" (Gullón 66).

25 In this assessment I differ from Chamberlin, who claims that, "Galdós' interest in the medical aspects of his first major named *ciego* [blind man, Pablo] is slight" (66).

26 The story is so remarkable that Scanlon characterizes it as a fairy tale, "In reality Teodoro is a rather idealized figure, and his story has a certain air of a fairy story," "En realidad Teodoro es una figura un tanto idealizada, y su historia tiene cierto aire

He describes the results of his examination of Pablo, "the ophthalmoscopic examination that I performed yesterday did not show me any retinal lesion or abnormality of the visual nerves"[27] He continues his assessment, "there is a fissure in the iris," hoping that he will find "the choroid and retina in a good condition" and not find "total blindness."[28] Galdós continues to employ ophthalmological terms in Golfín's explanation referring to the "vitreous humour" and to "glaucoma" and to "cortical layer" (159), indicating the extent of his preparatory study for the novel. The gelatinous substance between the lens of the eye and the retina (vitreous humour) and increased pressure within the eye potentially leading to blindness (glaucoma) were well-recognized at the time. Galdós's reference to a cortical layer, *capa cortical*, however, takes us to a controversy in brain physiology that became a burning topic among contemporary neurophysiologists. The Englishman David

---

de cuento de hadas" (88). Caudet remarks that, "the story of the Golfín brothers was not possible given the reality of Spain," "la novela de los Golfín no era possible en la realidad española" (*introducción* 43). Comparison with the subsequent experience of Marianela's companion, Felipe, in *El doctor Centeno* makes this abundantly clear.

27 'El examen catóptrico que hice ayer no me indica lesión retiniana ni alteración de los nervios de la visión' (*Marianela* 158). *Catóptrico* (Greek: *katoptron*=mirror), refers to an apparatus that permits an examination using reflected light and refers to the ophthalmoscope, a workable version of which was devised by Hermann von Helmholtz in 1851. A light source near the patient is reflected by a mirror close to the examining physician in the plane of the latter's gaze as he/she looks into the patient's eye. Galdós has studied the topic of cataracts and correctly identifies the crystalline lens as being opaque. More problematic, however, is the fact that if Pablo had no perception of light due to the density of his cataract, it would be because the cataract completely blocked the passage of light to the retina. This being so, light reflected by the *aparato catóptrico* would also be unable to penetrate to the back of the eye so that visual inspection of retina and optic nerve would be impossible.

28 "el iris tiene fisura;" "la coroides y la retina en buen estado;" "una amaurosis total" (*Marianela* 159). Fissure of the iris (otherwise known as a *coloboma*) is described as being associated with congenital cataracts (Deval 574). The choroid is the layer of blood vessels and connective tissue that lies between the outer coat of the eye (sclera) and the retina and is considered to supply the retina with oxygen. Complete *amaurosis* means "complete blindness." For the feasibility of examining the choroid in the presence of densely opaque congenital cataracts see the note above.

Ferrier had published findings in 1870s suggesting that visual function in the brain was localized to the superficial (cortical) layers of the lateral (parietal) aspects of the cerebral hemispheres. Independent work in Germany by Hermann Munk published in 1881, after the appearance of *Marianela*, suggested, in contrast, that visual cortical function was, in fact, located in the rear tips of the hemispheres (the occipital lobes). While it is doubtful that Galdós was aware of the details of the controversy, his reference to layers of the cerebral cortex, *capas corticales*, suggests that he knew about it at least in general outline.[29] Significantly, Galdós was also aware that optic atrophy could occur in the presence of cataracts, "in that republic of the eye there are many lazy elements that are atrophied,"[30] suggesting that he may have been aware that complete failure of light to reach and stimulate the retina until adult life was associated with impaired perception of light, even when the obstruction to light was removed. He later attributes Pablo's failure to see Golfín and Marianela to one side of him to loss of lateral vision that he associates with incomplete adaptation to sight, "still not having accustomed himself to the rotatory movement of the eye, he scarcely saw images to his side [...] seeing only that which lay in front of him."[31]

Galdós's litany of eye anatomy continues as he evokes Golfín's operative procedure with his reference to the hyaloid (*las hyaloides*), the posterior chamber of the eye (*la camera posterior*), the pupil (*contractilidad de la pupila*), the retina (*retina sensible*) and the optic nerve (*nervios llena de vida*) (*Marianela* 186–87).[32] Following the removal of bandages, Pablo's

29 The controversy of the 1870s and 1880s over the precise location of the visual cortex is described by Fishman. It was also the subject of a more contemporary review by the celebrated psychologist, William James in his *The Principles of Psychology*.

30 "en esa república del ojo, hay muchos holgazanes que se atrofian" (*Marianela* 158).

31 "No habiéndose familiarizado aún con los movimientos de rotación del ojo, apenas percibía las imágenes laterales [...] que solo veía lo que tenía delante" (*Marianela* 231).

32 Hyaloid canal: a small transparent canal running from the optic nerve disc to the lens of the eye; posterior chamber: a small space behind the iris but in front of the lens; pupil: aperture of variable size in the iris through which light enters the eye; retina: light sensitive layer of nerve cells at the back of the eye; optic nerve: at ophthalmoscopy, the optic disc is made up of retinal nerve fibres that pass backward from the eye to form the optic nerve, which is an extension of the brain.

sight is restored and with it comes an instant appreciation of visual aesthetics, "everything beautiful produces in him an enthusiasm bordering on delirium, all that is ugly causes him horror."[33]

This is the climactic event in *Marianela*. Many critical interpretations of the novel seem to take the miraculous restoration of Pablo's sight at face value, which is, no doubt, the author's intention. If so, the event must be accepted on a symbolic or metaphorical level since Pablo's sudden acquisition of visual acuity is utterly implausible. At the time that Galdós published *Marianela* in 1878, it had long been known that congenital cataracts needed to be removed in the first year of life if functional vision were to be achieved.[34] Subsequent studies of the development of the mammalian visual cortex in infancy have confirmed what was known empirically in Galdós's time, "innate mechanisms endow the visual system with highly specific connections, but visual experience early in life is necessary for their maintenance and full development."[35] In the human child, "Infantile cataract not only blurs the retinal image but also disrupts the development of visual pathways."[36] The first few months of life represent a phase of critical developmental such that, "Prior to and after these periods, the visual environment exerts a much weaker influence, hence the laboriously acquired visual functions of individuals who had their congenital cataracts removed late in life."[37] Ophthalmic texts of the time, available to Galdós's

33 "Todo lo que es bello le produce un entusiasmo que parece delirio; todo lo que es feo le causa horror" (*Marianela* 195).

34 Wecker advises in the treatment of congenital cataracts, "operate on children as soon as possible no matter how small they may be. Nothing damages sight more than the absence of normal visual function during the growth of the eye," "operad lo más pronto que posible á los niños por pequeños que sean. Nada deteriora más la visión que la ausencia de un funcionalismo regular durante el crecimiento del órgano de la vista" (318).

35 Wiesel 591.

36 Ondráček and Lokaj 95.

37 Breitmeyer 42. The English surgeon William Cheselden reported in 1728 the treatment of congenital cataracts by the traditional method of posterior dislocation of the lens, *couching*, in a 14-year-old boy. After 14 years of blindness, the lad had great difficulty in recognizing the size and shape of objects that he knew well by touch. He could not recall how to distinguish a dog from a cat by sight, but recognized the

medical friends if not to the author himself, clearly state the importance of the removal of congenital cataracts in infancy if loss of vision, nystagmus and squint are to be avoided.[38] Given the study of ophthalmology that Galdós undertook in preparation for *Marianela* it seems highly likely that he was aware of this literal impossibility but chose to disregard it in order to preserve the integrity of his story.

A related improbability is Pablo's instant grasp of the conventional visual aesthetics of his age. In real life, a previously completely blind subject whose vision is restored in adult life, if he or she is not actually blind, has difficulty in coming to terms with visual experience and making sense of the images he or she sees. Pablo's immediate ability to distinguish the features of the beautiful woman from those of the ugly owes more to a Platonic idea of an innate sense of form than it does to human physiology.[39] Similarly the constant equivalence of the visual with "reality" may owe something to Plato's metaphor of the cave in *The Republic* and bears such truth as it has to philosophical rather than empirical considerations. Taking the symbolic story in its own terms, Pablo's acquisition of sight is accompanied by complete blindness to the reality of his relationship with Marianela, in his enthusiasm to marry his cousin Florentina. For this parent-mediated match not only enables him to establish himself in the bourgeois, patriarchal hierarchy of his time but also serves to reunite the formerly divided Faustino inheritance. The insistence throughout the novel of reality as visual must be symbolic rather than literal, since an important part of Pablo's reality before surgery is non-visual and no less real for that.[40] The reality that the caring Teodoro laments, as he sees Marianela slip

---

latter instantly when he felt its coat. After picking up a cat, "he was observ'd to look at her steadfastly, and then setting her down, said 'So Puss! I shall know you another Time'" (448).

38 For example Deval 576–77 cites an 18-year-old who, on removal of congenital cataracts, was found to have very poor vision due to optic nerve atrophy. See also Meyer 404.

39 Montesinos also makes this observation (*I* 238).

40 The tradition of the blind seeing a reality that the sight-enabled do not goes back to Classical times. Galdós continues this tradition in Lucía in *Ángel Guerra* and Almudena in *Misericordia*.

away before his eyes, appears to be confined to the visual. A more broadly considered reality might view Pablo as an impulsive, shallow young man whose character belies the Platonic perfection of his handsome features that so fascinates onlookers.[41]

Teodoro Golfín recurs in another novel of Galdós, *La de Bringas*, where loss of sight is a dominant theme. Francisco Bringas works as a minor functionary in the Royal Palace in Madrid, where he also lives with his family. He occupies his leisure hours by making an excruciatingly fine and detailed hair portrait as a memorial gift to his friends, the Pez family, who have recently lost a daughter. The effort of focusing on such minute work is too much for him and he suffers an attack of blindness cured only by weeks of slow recovery from inflammation of the conjunctiva.[42] This condition causes light to irritate the eyes, *photophobia*, requiring treatment by rest and protection of the eyes from light with bandages. This enforced blindness enables his wife, Rosalía, to conceal from her cost-conscious husband her pawning of family valuables to pay for her passion for fashionable clothes. As Bringas' vision slowly improves, Rosalía becomes the prey of money lenders and finally has to resort to a future of genteel prostitution in order to redeem the valuables whose absence she can no longer conceal. Meanwhile, greater events in Spanish society, unheeded by the Bringas family, have taken place and culminate in the September Revolution of 1868. As Queen Isabel flees the palace, Bringas refuses to compromise with the new order, as a result of which he and his family have to move to humbler quarters. The novel ends with Rosalía as the remaining support of the family, facing her newly discovered role as courtesan.

Early in the novel, Francisco Bringas is warned that he is heading for trouble when he experiences double vision and giddiness after a session

41 One recalls the similar effortlessness with which that other witty, handsome, young man, Juanito Santa Cruz, slides into matrimony with Jacinta Cordero in *Fortunata y Jacinta*. The two *señoritos* seem to have in common a talent for forgetting their previous commitments to working-class girls.

42 Conjunctiva: "the mucous membrane that covers the front of the eye and lines the inside of the eyelids" (OED).

at his desk (130).[43] Not long afterwards he abruptly loses his sight. In the family distress that follows, a friend of the family, Cándida, quotes an anecdote that ophthalmic migraine, *jaqueca oftálmica*, can produce such symptoms and that they can be expected to be transient (148).[44] An elderly physician is summoned and makes a different diagnosis of retinal congestion, *congestión retiniana*, and prescribes strict rest, bandaging of the eyes, a *derivativo* and a tranquilizing medication to help him sleep at night (149).[45] Though Bringas suffers severe headaches and pain in the eyes that night, the physician reassures him, when he returns, that his affliction will resolve with time and patience.

Bringas' impatience gets the better of him, however, and he cannot resist the temptation to lift the bandage to test his perception of light. Though he finds that he is no longer blind, light still irritates his eyes and is associated with visual spectra (abnormal images before the eyes), "thousands of points of light or of thin, metallic rays [of light], moveable and fleeting images of the accursed hairs [...] retained by the retina."[46] A week passes with little change in the light-induced pain despite compresses of belladonna that Rosalía is instructed to place over his eyes, together with the belladonna and laudanum that she rubs into his temples. To this regime opium and calomel are added at night (159).[47]

43 Page references are from the Cátedra edition of *La de Bringas* edited by Alda Blanco and Carlos Blanco Aguinaga, hereafter cited as *Bringas*.

44 *jaqueca oftálmica* was so-called because of the frequency of visual symptoms that accompanied the (usually) one-sided headaches. Galdós suffered from this condition and appears to have studied it in pages that he marked in one of the two monographs sent him by the Catalán neurologist, Armangué y Tuset.

45 A *derivativo* is a medication intended to draw to the surface fluids that have accumulated causing congestion (*Diccionario de la Lengua Española* 1925). *Congestión retiniana* (also *rétinite séreuse*) appears in contemporary ophthalmic texts (del Toro *I* 719; Deval 652 ff.; Meyer 305 ff.).

46 "millares de puntos luminosos o de tenues rayos metálicos, movibles, fugaces, imagines de los malditos [...] pelos que conservaba la retina" (*Bringas* 156).

47 Cold compresses over the eyes are recommended by Meyer (312). Belladonna was applied externally for complaints involving superficial structures (Hirtz 754). Both Hirtz and Buignet appear to suggest that there were few conditions at the time

Despite the unnamed physician's promises of a rapid recovery (163–64), Bringas' condition drags on and he is still not well enough to take even a limited stroll (172). After transient improvement, symptoms get worse again and the physician is hard-pressed to account for the failure of his treatment (197), and can only recommend more rest and protection of the eyes from light. The family's frequent visitor, Manuel Pez, comes to the conclusion that they have avoided when he observes that the doctor has no specialist knowledge of eye disease, "I don't know why you didn't call an oculist on the first day ... This good fellow [...] it seems to me, knows as much about eyes as a mole."[48] With his sight deteriorating further, Bringas finally yields to the pressure of his wife and Pez such that, when the hapless physician finally confesses himself out of his depth, Bringas accepts his recommendation of the most highly regarded oculist in Madrid, Teodoro Golfín (201).

Upon arrival, Golfín immediately takes command of the situation diagnosing "a little conjunctivitis."[49] He dispenses with the multiplicity of medications prescribed by his predecessor, recommending only atropine and rest. He prophesies confidently, "you will see" though adds rather

for which belladonna (or its purified element, Atropine) were not recommended. Treatments for epilepsy, neuralgia, insanity, tetanus and asthma all had their advocates, though its use for dilatation of the pupil and for relief of ocular pain has best stood the test of time. Laudanum is an alcoholic tincture of opiate alkaloids that was popularized by the English physician Thomas Sydenham in the 1660s and became an ingredient of a wide range of medicines in the XVIII and XIX centuries (Hodgson 45–77). Its use in Bringas' case would have been to relieve pain and to promote sleep.

Calomelano (calomel, mercurous chloride) rivalled atropine in the number of conditions for which it was prescribed, despite its long-term toxicity. Meyer recommends it for both "parenchymatous" and syphilitic retinitis (312–15).

48 "Yo no sé cómo desde el primer día no llamaron ustedes a un oculista ... Este buen señor [...] me parece a mí que entiende tanto de ojos como un topo" (*Bringas* 197).

49 "Hay un poco de conjunctivitis" (*Bringas* 202). Unobtrusively here, Galdós demonstrates his study of ophthalmology. The anonymous doctor has been treating Bringas for retinitis, that is, disease at the *back* of the eye, whereas the renowned oculist, Golfín, undertakes a successful course of treatment based on a diagnosis of a disease affecting the *front* of the eye, conjunctivitis.

mysteriously, "you will see what you have never seen before" (202). Golfín cauterizes Bringas's eyes three times a week with a paintbrush dipped in silver nitrate followed by the application of a solution of common salt, followed by a cold compress (211).[50] This is followed by such improvement after twelve days that Golfín is able to prophesy complete cure in a matter of weeks. The cauterization regime is changed to copper sulphate and Bringas is permitted to remove the protective bandaging while in a darkened room. Progress is steady and he is allowed out of the home while wearing protective dark glasses and a green eyeshade.

All seems well until news of the September Revolution breaks. Bringas then suffers a severe reverse that leaves him not only with recurring visual symptoms but also, more troublingly, difficulty with speech and gait. This suggests a mild stroke as a result of altered blood flow to his dominant cerebral dominant hemisphere including the area of the brain responsible for speech. Galdós includes details of his visual hallucinations, "and [his] visual organs had got up to their old tricks, altering and colouring objects in an extraordinary manner."[51] Such visual hallucinations of colour suggest damage to the visual pathways at the back of the brain such as can follow reduced blood flow.[52] Even as Galdós has us bid farewell to the failing Bringas at the end of the novel, it would seem that he cannot resist the temptation to include a subtlety from his medical repertoire to enhance the authenticity of his story.

50 Such painting of the conjunctiva with silver nitrate is recommended by Meyer when the increased blood flow to the area has become chronic. Immediately after cauterization, any excess is washed away with a solution of common salt. Copper sulphate cauterization was an alternative. For the sensation of heat that followed the process, a cold compress was recommended (50–51).

51 "y el órgano de la visión había vuelto a sus antiguas mañas, alterando y coloreando de un modo extraño los objetos" (*Bringas* 295).

52 The variety of visual hallucinations as a result of alterations of the central visual pathways (nerve tracts in the brain) has been described more recently by Vaphiades *et al.* It was also known to neurologists of Galdós's time, however, exemplified by Armangué y Tuset's description of visual hallucinations seen in the context of ocular migraine (*Estudios* 157–63). Galdós may well have been drawing on his own experience of the latter condition, which he suffered in the course of many years.

CHAPTER 7

Childhood Diseases

Child mortality in Spain was appalling, above all, among abandoned infants at foundlings' hospitals. Tolosa Latour quotes an overall mortality in 1859 of 50%, though in one institution, *La Inclusa*, it rose to 85%. In contrast, he found that newborns looked after in homes of wet-nurses had a mortality 14% (*Niño* 88). In a 5-year period in the 1890s, Hauser found that over 24% of live births failed to reach the age of one year.[1] The vulnerability of the young is further underlined by the finding that between 1860 and 1900, "children under the age of six never comprised more than about 12% of Madrid's total population, yet consistently accounted for more than 40% of the deaths in the city."[2]

Confronting this mortality, Tolosa Latour distinguished himself as a paediatric clinician and author of books on childhood disease. He also laboured to promote national legislation (*La ley Tolosa*) for the physical and moral protection of children under the age of ten years.[3] In 1881, Tolosa published, "The medical care of abandoned children," *La protección médica al niño desválido*. In the same year, Galdós exposed the national scandal of child labour in his description of Mariano, *Pecado*, the brother of Isidora Rufete in *La desheredada*, labouring mindlessly for long hours in the treadmill of a rope-making factory doing, "work [...] fit for mules."[4] Galdós expresses admiration for Tolosa Latour and his profession in the prologue to Tolosa's collection of stories about childhood:

1 *Madrid I* 542.
2 Goldman 208.
3 Sánchez and Guijarro 126–27.
4 "trabajo [...] para mulos" (*desheredada* 108).

> I must tell you specifically that I shall always admire the medical specialty that you have chosen, as you establish yourself in the profession, because caring for sick little ones seems to me to be of the greatest distinction and difficulty of that caring and experimental science. The patience and courage that it requires, the demanding nature of the work, and the extremely sad exposure to human misery, transform it into a kind of chivalry both scientific and religious.[5]

Galdós loved children and declared as much.[6] His friend and later his physician, Gregorio Marañón, observed that, while he was shy with adults and detested public display, he related well to children. Marañón describes his own experience as a child when Galdós would play with him for long periods sharing private games and stories.[7] Other contemporaries commented on Galdós's special affection for children and his ability to relate to them.[8] Galdós must have observed children not only at play but in the classroom for he also studied the ideas of the most enlightened educators of his day. These included the theories of Pestalozzi that emphasized the ability of children to learn through spontaneous observation, intuition and play. Others were those of Froebel, who extended Pestalozzi's practice that

5 "Me concreto á decirte que admiré siempre la especialidad profesional que has escogido, porque cuidar á los pequeñuelos enfermos me parece la mayor gloria y la dificultad más grande de esa ciencia experimental y caritativa, que al erigirse en profesión, por la paciencia y valor que exige, por la rudeza del trabajo, y su contacto tristísimo con la miseria humana, viene á convertirse en una especie de caballería entre científica y religiosa" (*Prólogo* iii–iv).

6 "the most interesting part of humanity, the younsters, who I like so much, as you know, and with whom I get on so well," "a parte más interesante de la humanidad, los chiquillos, que á mí me gustan tanto, como sabes, y con los cuales hago muy buenas migas" (*Prólogo* iii).

7 "But with children, such as I, he used to relax in abundant and happy chatter, full of witty childishness, mixed with the experiences, full of humour, of his great and profound life," "Mas con los niños, como yo, se explayaba en una verborrea copiosa y alegre, llena de graciosas puerilidades, mezcladas con la experiencia, llena de humor, de su vasta y profunda vida" (*Menéndez* 437).

8 Summarized by Shoemaker, "But Galdós loved them [children] all [...] The common touch that don Benito possessed was seen especially in his relations with little folk," "Pero Galdós los quería a todos [...] El don de gentes que poseía do Benito se veía muy especialmente en sus relaciones con la gente menuda" (*Cómo* 13).

took into account the stages of childhood development. Froebel employed the horticultural metaphor in his *Kindergartens* where children could grow as they developed manual and scholastic skills. Galdós was, perhaps, influenced in this by Tolosa Latour who devotes a chapter on infant education in *El Niño* in which he praises the educational ideas of Rousseau, Pestalozzi, Froebel and Herbert Spencer. Galdós makes an ironic plea for humane and constructive teaching in *El doctor Centeno* in the character of Jesús Delgado, a visionary obsessed with educational reform, who is driven mad by his dismissal after 20 years of service at the *Dirección de Instrucción Pública*. Galdós intensifies his criticism by describing in *El doctor Centeno* the crushing effect of traditional rote learning under threat of physical punishment that Felipe Centeno has to endure in Pedro Polo's school.[9] Galdós also portrays children in the streets of Madrid's shabbier suburbs. As an example, he records street life in his description of Felipe Centeno and his school friends as they play at bullfighting. A grimmer location is the setting of gang warfare of street urchins in *La desheredada* in which the 13-year-old *Pecado* stabs another boy to death taking a momentous step in a criminal career that will end on the scaffold.

At the same time Galdós's clinical eye sought medical features that would augment his naturalistic description. In addition to recording the scanty clothes, malnutrition and filth of the urchins playing at street warfare, he assesses their medical conditions, "inherited rickets imprinted with its yellow stamp the multitude of heads, inscribing their predestination to crime."[10] *Raquitismo heredado* was a poorly defined entity in Galdós's time since not only was the underlying cause not known but the term was sometimes used simply to mean "sickly" or "weakly." It was also linked with other conditions such as tuberculosis and scrofula,[11] while Joseph Parrot, a leading Paris paediatrician of the day, affirmed that all childhood rickets was syphilitic in origin.[12] Rickets was recognized as being associated with

9 *Centeno* 153–62.

10 "El raquitismo heredado marcaba con su sello amarillo multitud de cabezas, inscribiendo la predestinación del crimen" (*desheredada* 149).

11 Lannelongue 379.

12 Parrot, *Rachitis* 35–40, 57.

poverty and poor hygiene and was particularly common in children reared in dark, damp and cold dwellings, although it could also be seen in the young of the well-to-do. Malnutrition was recognized as being related to rickets, and a good diet and sea bathing were recommended for those fortunate enough to be taken to the coast.[13] The consumption of fish oils is described by Lannelongue, quoting Trousseau, as a folk remedy long practised in the cloudier climes of Holland and Britain.[14] It is unlikely, however, that ragamuffins such as those described by Galdós would ever receive it.

That Galdós goes on to relate the urchins' *raquitismo heredado* to a future in crime reflects an aspect of biological determinism common in his age. Crime was related to poverty and disease by social physicians and, since it ran in families, it was often presumed to be a form of inherited degeneration. While hygienists like Monlau saw the alleviation of poverty as a remedy for this degeneration,[15] Galdós expresses faith in the power of education to avoid raising generations of criminals.[16] He sees little hope, however, for this band in the *plazuela de las Peñuelas*, "they were the discord of the future, a growing part of Spain to come, such that if measles, smallpox, fevers and rickets did not eliminate them [...] they

13 Tolosa Latour translated from the French a text by Andrés-Théodore Brochard on the value of sea bathing for sick children in 1893. He was also instrumental in the foundation, with the Franciscan Padre Lerchundi, of Spain's first seaside sanitarium for rickety and tuberculous children at Chipiona in the province of Cádiz. Galdós supported the enterprise by donating to it the proceeds of a charity performance of *El abuelo* in 1904 (Ricard).

14 "Trousseau [...] points out that in England and Holland, from time immemorial, [...] the common folk have been in the habit of giving fish oil to their rickety children," "Trousseau [...] nos montre que, de temps immémorial, en Angleterre, en Hollande [...] les gens du peuple avaient l'habitude de donner des huiles de poisson à leurs enfants rachitiques" (599). In fact, fish oil already appears to have gained medical sanction, since it is referred to by Routh (498). Scientific proof of the role of dietary deficiency as a cause of rickets, and the discovery of vitamin D, abundant in fish oil, had to wait until the twentieth century.

15 *Remedios.*

16 The prologue to *La desheredada* is dedicated by Galdós to the teachers of Spain as the true healers of the country's social ills.

would, perhaps, become men of account and, without doubt, vagabonds and criminals."[17] The distinction between heredity and environment was largely moot, however, since it was widely assumed at the time that the influence of adverse physical and moral circumstances in parents would be transmitted to their children by biological inheritance.[18]

In listing measles, smallpox, fever and rickets for which the street urchins were at risk, Galdós takes it for granted that uncontrolled infectious fevers of childhood, such as whooping cough, diphtheria, croup and typhus, could be expected to cull a significant proportion of every generation. The well-to-do might move their families to new premises temporarily to try to escape epidemics of whooping cough and measles, as Galdós describes in *León Roch*, but for the poor there was nothing for it but to stay put and take their chances.[19] For them, conditions in the poorer suburbs, *barrios*, of Madrid, such as those on the incline facing south toward the river Manzanares: *Inclusa, Hospital* and *Latina* were extremely unhealthy.[20] Having few sewers, they had to cope with outdoor latrines, *pozos negros*, and the accumulation of waste of all kinds in the streets. In these areas of the city, mortality from diphtheria/croup reached a peak in 1886, and was then more lethal than scarlet fever, measles, whooping cough or typhus.[21] An epidemiological study of the time indicates that Madrid's mortality from diphtheria was higher than in any other of the thirty largest cities in Western Europe.[22]

Even the well-to-do were obliged to see their children run the gauntlet of mortal disease and to accept with resignation the loss of many of them.

17 "Eran la discordia del porvenir, una parte crecida de la España futura, tal que si no la quitaran el sarampión, las viruelas, las fiebres y el raquitismo, [...] que saldrían quizás hombres de provecho y sin duda vagos y criminales" (*desheredada* 150).

18 Hauser, *siglo* 344.

19 *La familia de León Roch*. Ed. Íñigo Sánchez Llama. Madrid: Cátedra, 2003. 371. Hereafter cited as *Roch*.

20 High mortality rates in these *barrios* in the 1890s in comparison with other *distritos municipals* are recorded by Hauser, *Madrid I* 531–32.

21 Tolosa Latour, *Instrucciones* 16.

22 Monmeneu 104.

This is reflected by Galdós in *Fortunata y Jacinta* in which he describes the family of Isabel Cordero where only her "prodigious fecundity" managed to outrun losses from infectious disease. Of her seventeen live children, "that packed crop was thinned out by diphtheria and scarlet fever and in 1870 only nine remained. The first two died soon after birth and, after a while, an older child was lost thinning the ranks [...] three died at four-month intervals. Those who passed the age of ten grew normally."[23]

So aware was Galdós of the diseases of childhood that they enter his writing as metaphors of adult life. Measles' contagiousness and inevitability were such that Juanito's mother in *Fortunata y Jacinta* could look upon her son's nocturnal adventures with women of the lower classes as being no more than a passing phase to be expected of one of his generation, "it is the measles from which no youth of these times is immune."[24] When Juanito obsessively searches the more disreputable quarters of Madrid looking for Fortunata and exhausts himself to the point of catching pneumonia, he is, "seeking the cure for the typhus of curiosity that consumed him."[25]

Galdós provides a more literal image of typhus in his description of the death of Paco Ramos, *Posturitas*, witnessed by his schoolfellow, Luís Cadalso, in *Miau*:

> Posturitas had been terribly delirious all night and for part of the morning. At that moment he was quieter still without a return of his high temperature [...] he glanced at his friends with an astonished and glassy gaze. Although his eyes were inflamed they had a deathly look, his lips were so purple that they seemed black and there were wine-red blotches in his cheeks [...] the fixed and lacklustre gaze of his schoolfellow made him tremble. No doubt Paco Ramos was unable to recognize the three

23 "El garrotillo y la escarlatina fueron entresacando aquella mies apretada, y en 1870 no quedaban ya más que nueve. Los dos primeros volaron a poco de nacidos. De tiempo en tiempo se moría uno, ya crecidito, y se aclaraban las filas [...] se murieron tres con intervalo de cuatro meses. Los que rebasaron de los diez años, se iban criando regularmente" (*Fortunata I* 156).

24 "Es un sarampión de que no se libra ningún muchacho de estos tiempos" (*Fortunata I* 191).

25 "buscando remedio al tifus de curiosidad que le consumía" (*Fortunata I*, 442).

> except for Luisito, because he only said *Miau, Miau,* after which his head collapsed on the pillow.[26]

The next time that Luís sees him is when the dead boy has been laid out, "his face very yellow with purple blotches, the mouth half open and almost black," which the poor visitor finds terrifying.[27]

In the vivid style inherent in Naturalist writing, Galdós here portrays the grimness of acute disease in this, one of his many studies of dying. He leads us into the sick room of *Posturitas* and gives us such a detailed description of one of the forms of typhus that it seems highly likely that he had witnessed something similar himself. A contemporary text describes three forms of the disease that could only be distinguished clinically, in the absence of any available laboratory studies for confirmation. Abdominal typhus is dominated by gastrointestinal symptoms and can be confused with the enteritis of typhoid fever, a disease that was also endemic in Madrid. The central nervous form of typhus preferentially attacks the brain producing rapid descent into coma. In contrast, Galdós characterizes *Posturitas*' disease, with its intermittent fever and delirium, its blotchy rash and its inflammation of the eyes, as belonging to the epidemic type that was recognized as being associated with crowded and unhygienic living conditions.[28] This disease killed thousands in Madrid every year and treatment could only be supportive since there was no cure and the responsible organism was unknown.

26 "*Posturitas* había delirado atrozmente toda la noche y parte de la mañana. En aquel momento estaba más tranquilo, sin que el recargo se iniciara aún. [...] Echo a sus amigos una mirada atónita y vidriosa. Tenía los ojos, aunque inflamados, mortecinos, los labios tan cárdenos que parecían negros, y en los pómulos manchados de color de vino [...] La mirada fija y sin luz de su compañero de escuela le hacía temblar. Paco Ramos sin duda no conoció de los tres más que a Luisito; porque sólo dijo *Miau, Miau*, después de lo cual su cabeza se derrumbó sobre la almohada" (*Miau* 275, author's italics).

27 "la cara muy amarilla, con manchas moradas, lo boca entreabierta y un tono casi negro" (*Miau*, 303).

28 This classification of typhus appears in volume 3 of Jaccoud's *Tratado de patología interna* (565–66), a copy of which was in Galdós's library, bearing a dedication to him by Tolosa Latour.

The croup and diphtheria that Galdós mentions were often considered at the time as the same condition, in spite of the fact that the milder condition ("croup," "false croup,") had been described earlier in the century.[29] Another name for the disease, *garrotillo*, is related to that other means of fatal asphyxiation, the *garrote*, by which condemned felons met their end on the scaffold. Galdós provides a vivid account of croup/diphtheria in *La familia de León Roch* where León watches Monina succumb to the disease. He shivers with terror to see Monina:

> with her face distorted and livid with lips violet in colour, eyes wide open blinking and tearful, her neck stiff and tightly swollen with enlarged lymph nodes. [León] suffered even more to hear her laboured moaning that was neither cough nor speech, but something resembling the voice of a ventriloquist, a heart-rending sharp sound as disturbing as the screech of a whistle in a demon's mouth and resembling the inflection of a cock's crow [...] He saw her contract in suffocation, burying her fingers in her neck anxious to pierce it to allow the flow of needed air to her obstructed throat. A terrible sight! The death of a child by strangulation [...] with the convulsions of a hung criminal and the terror of asphyxia is one of the cruellest examples of the inexorable anguish, whether by trial or punishment, that accompanies human life.[30]

29 The milder "false croup" or "stridulous laryngitis" (now viral laryngo-tracheo-branchitis) was first differentiated from diphtheria by Bretonneau in 1826 (Rolleston 6). Though "true" diphtheria was endemic throught Europe in Galdós's day, it had been responsible for lethal epidemics since the sixteenth century interspersed by intervals in which it seemed to disappear completely. It was responsible for a severe epidemic in Spain around 1581 when, under the names of *qarrotillo* or *morbus suffocans*, it became well-known. Loeffler in 1884 was the first to isolate the bacterium that causes diphtheria and to grow it in pure culture. In 1886–87 he succeeded in isolating diphtheria toxin that produces the disease (Loeffler 28, 35). Antiserum to protect against the toxin was developed in the 1890s (48–52).

30 "con la cara lívida y descompuesta, los labios violados, los ojos muy abiertos, pestañeantes y lagrimosos, el cuello entumecido, tirante, hinchado por el infarto de los ganglios, y padeció más al oír aquel gemido estertoroso, que no era tos ni habla, sino algo semejante a voz de ventrílocuo, una nota aguda, desgarradora, agria como chirrido de un pito en boca de un demonio y parecida a la inflexión del canto de un gallo [...] La vio contraerse sofocada, llevándose los dedos al cuello para clavárselos, con ansia de agujerearse para dar paso al aire que faltaba a su garganta obstruida. ¡Espectáculo horrible! La muerte de un niño por estrangulación [...] con las convulsiones del

This depiction has the immediacy of being written by one who had seen the condition firsthand. Indeed, Galdós once said as much when he wrote that in order to be able to write about something, "I don't want anyone to tell me about what I can see it with my own eyes and touch with my own hands."[31] Consistent with this, there is more of individual experience in this description than would be found in a purely clinical text. Croup/diphtheria had a mortality of 77% at the time and the number of deaths recorded in Madrid had risen from 242 in 1880 to 1,360 in 1885.[32] While the diphtheria bacillus was identified in 1884, a specific antitoxin was not available until 1895 and treatment could usually be only supportive. Bretonneau had performed the first tracheotomy for diphtheria in an adult in 1826,[33] but the operation was more difficult in small children, the majority of those affected, and was frequently fatal due to complicating infection.[34] The alternative, intubation with a tube entering the larynx through the mouth or nose, which was able to relieve the laryngeal blockage that obstructed breathing, was not developed until 1889, well after *La familia de León Roch* was published.[35] For a child reaching the extreme of Monina's condition, the experienced physician could only echo Moreno Rubio's lament, "there's no hope," *No hay esperanza* (337).

Contemporary physicians managed as best they could. Tolosa Latour, probably responding to a recent epidemic that he saw in his work at the *Hospital de Niño Jesús* where he was on the staff, wrote a popular information sheet for the Spanish Society of Hygiene in 1886. This informed parents about the best measures to help them avoid infection in their children, with

criminal ahorcado y el espanto de la asfixia, es uno de los más crueles ejemplos del dolor inexorable que acompaña, como prueba o castigo, a la vida humana" (*Roch* 336).

31 "No me gusta que nadie me cuente lo que puedo ver con mis ojos y tocar con mis manos" *(Prensa* 18 Dec. 1893)

32 Marco 26.

33 Rolleston 4.

34 Gelfand 1.

35 O'Dwyer 299–303. Bouchut had proposed endotracheal intubation for diphtheria in Paris in 1855, but his idea failed to gain official sanction (O'Dwyer 266).

advice for appropriate nursing for those who developed the disease.[36] He warns readers of the high mortality of diphtheria and although he mentions tracheotomy, the technique of making an aperture in the windpipe below laryngeal obstruction then occasionally applied to adults with diphtheria, he does not mention its use to infants in this text. Later, however, Tolosa does appear to have performed the operation himself, and it was being performed more widely in France.[37]

Galdós portrays a different infectious disease of childhood in the demise of Torquemada's prodigy-son, Valentín, who dies of acute meningitis in *Torquemada en la hoguera*. Galdós has Valentín, the pride of Torquemada's life, come home from school with a high fever and drowsiness that does not resemble that of normal sleep. The son-in-law, Dr Quevedo, who is immediately summoned, recognizes the seriousness of Valentín's condition and advises that the boy needs relief from all his intellectual labours and needs to recover in the rough tranquillity of the country. In so doing he expresses the prevailing belief, found in a text belonging to Galdós, that excess mental fatigue is one of the factors that predisposes to acute meningitis.[38]

Valentín is described as having an astonished expression, with the sparkling eyes that are described in the first stage of the disease. In this phase there is typically cerebral excitation associated with severe and unrelenting headache. However, as he lapses into the delirium that is typical of the second phase, his speech is halting and ideas incoherent. As the delirium deepens, Galdós describes a fearful look in Valentín's eyes and spasms of the muscles as if he were jumping in his bed, a feature listed in a contemporary description of the disease. More disturbing still is the shrill meningitic cry, "like the squawk of a peacock,"[39] that rings through the house as Valentín's respiration becomes increasingly difficult, his delirium deepens and his high fever consumes him, despite all treatment. The latter consists of the

36 *Instrucciones* 1886.
37 García Almansa 29.
38 Jaccoud, *I* 425.
39 "semejante al alarido del pavo real" (*hoguera* 46).

application of cooling ice to the head and counter-irritants to the scalp and other parts of the body, both measures also referred to in Jaccoud's medical text (*I* 433). In Valentín's final moments, Galdós has him cry that angels are calling for him, in response to which his father suffers an epileptic convulsion and loses consciousness. It is not clear whether Galdós had witnessed death from acute meningitis first hand, but the vividness and detail of his description strongly suggest that he had.

Galdós assembles similar detail in his depiction of the death of Ción, the adored and beautiful six-year old daughter of Ángel in *Ángel Guerra*. At first she develops a high fever for which no obvious cause is identified. Her native intelligence and imagination appear accentuated by this temperature for she demands to be told fabulous stories for, "her mind burned as did her blood, and from that heat sprang like sparks ideas and strings of stories of extraordinary originality."[40] These stories seem so imaginatively heightened that they suggest the development of early delirium since her compulsive chatter is difficult to calm, even when she is bribed with the promise of toys to be quiet. Only occasionally does she lapse into a drowsiness that brings home to her father the terrifying realization that her condition may be mortal. Just as Torquemada tries to bargain for the life of his son by reforming his life with Christian good works, Ángel undertakes to renounce his former revolutionary fervour, and in addition, offers the life of his sick mistress, Dulcenombre, in a sacrificial exchange for the recovery of his daughter. After a brief respite, however, Ción's fever and increased heart rate return with a vengeance, unresponsive to all treatment, causing her doctor, Augusto Miquis, to warn that the condition is becoming dangerous. She starts to roll her eyes and to adopt a provocative and suggestive expression inappropriate for a child. Revealing his medical knowledge, Galdós refers to Ción's expression as an "unusual look that is technically known as *cynical*".[41] Despite cold compresses applied to the head and body, the fever advances and Ción adopts unusual, extreme and asym-

40 "Su mente ardía, lo mismo que su sangre de aquel rescoldo brotaban como chispas conceptos y retahílas anecdóticas de peregrine originalidad" (*Guerra* 162).

41 "mirada singular que técnicamente se llama *cínica*" (*Guerra* 172, author's italics).

metrical facial expressions culminating in a major convulsion. Desperate friction rubs of her entire body offer the child no relief and she dies with a "sardonic smile" on her face.[42] Ángel is submerged in incapacitating grief while Ción's governess, Leré, responds to the tragedy with a convulsion, as Torquemada did to his.

The extreme vividness of this episode suggests strongly that Galdós had seen a similar scene, elaborated though it is with details of Ción's hyperactive imagination. The apparent lack of diagnosis of the cause of Ción's fever reflects a contemporary difficulty, beyond the clinical examination, in determining a fever's cause. "Fever" alone could be considered as a disease in its own right and so identified as a cause of death.[43] Galdós's repeated reference to Ción's temperature partly reflects the contemporary influence of measurement-based *physiopathological* medicine, in this case with the clinical thermometer, then a recent development.[44] The pulse rate and the changes in composition of the urine were similarly regarded as having a great prognostic significance. The treatment regime of cold compresses, digitalis and friction rubs to the body, however, give an idea of how slender was the range of therapeutic resources then available to treat Ción's disease.

A detailed reading of Galdós's description, however, suggests that he may have had a more specific disease in mind. For in addition to describing an uncontrollably high temperature and racing pulse, he adds that Ción suffers from spasm of the facial muscles producing a most unusual *cynical* expression that is quite unlike that of a normal child. In addition, he describes her rolling herself up into a ball,[45] remaining otherwise in a

42 "sonreír sardónico" (*Guerra* 175).

43 The first volume of Jaccoud's *Tratado de patología interna* devotes a chapter (VII) to a discussion of fever, much of it, seemingly, as an independent disease, illustrated by colour plates of temperature graphs.

44 For a discussion of this *physiopathological* phase in XIX c. medicine, see Laín Entralgo 375 ff. Also J.M.S Pearce, "A brief history of the clinical thermometer." For thermometry in Spain see José María López Piñero, "El saber médico en la sociedad española del siglo XIX," in José María López Piñero, Luís García Ballester and Pilar Faus Sevilla, 102.

45 "she was completely curled up like a ball," "toda ella se hizo un ovillo" (*Guerra* 173).

mentally clear, hyper-excited state, until she finally suffers from a convulsion. The last key feature given by Galdós is that Ción is described as having the grimace of a *sardonic smile*.[46] In Galdós's time, there were two conditions primarily associated with this unusual feature, one was poisoning with strychnine and the other was tetanus.[47] Reference to Galdós's edition of Jaccoud's *Tratado* reveals a description that includes distorting facial spasms, "the contraction [of the muscles of the face] is sufficient to pull the features of the face to its margins".[48] Typical of tetanus is the unremittingly high temperature with preserved mental clarity not seen in meningitis, the condition with which it could be confused, "Cerebral function remains intact until depressed respiration produces asphyxia, but the TEMPERATURE and the circulation are abnormal from the first stages of the disease."[49] In addition there can be spasm of the trunk of the body in forward flexion in which the body curls up into a ball, though this is less common than the classical, backward hyperextension, "the body [...] remains curved either backwards (*opisthotonos*), which is the most common, or curled forwards (*emprosthotonos*)."[50]

46 "disordered expression of that sardonic smile with which she left this life," "expresión descompuesta y de aquel sonreír sardónico con que se despidió la vida" (*Guerra* 175). The earliest use of "sardonic" in English in a medical context is listed by the OED as 1822, "The nostrils are drawn upward, and the cheeks backwards toward the ears, so that the whole countenance assumes the air of a cynic spasm or sardonic grin."

47 The latter had a certain topicality in 1891, when Ángel Guerra was published, since Arthur Nicolaier had identified *Clostridium tetani*, the responsible bacterium, in samples of soil as recently as 1884. In that same year, Carle and Rattone produced the disease in animals by injecting them with pus from a patient who had died of the disease. In 1889 the organism was grown in pure culture for the first time by Kitasato Shibasaburo (Udwadia 2). Tetanus toxin was isolated by Faber in 1890, while antitoxin was isolated and used therapeutically for the first time in the early 1890s (4).

48 "su contracción [los músculos de la cara] es suficiente para distender hacía la periferia las facciones del rostro" (*I* 776).

49 "Las funciones cerebrales permanecen intactas hasta que el entorpecimiento de la respiración produce el estado asfítico; pero la CALORIFACION y la circulación están perturbadas desde las primeras fases de la enfermedad" (*I* 778, author's capitals).

50 "el cuerpo [...] permanence doblado, ya hacía atrás (*opistótonos*), que es lo más frecuente, ya hacía adelante (*emprostótonos*)" (*I* 777, author's italics).

The long entry on tetanus by Poncet de Cluny comments that the hyperpyrexia to 42–43° of the disease is one of the most extreme fevers known, "the temperature reaches the highest degrees known, 42°, 43°."[51] This unusual coexistence of high temperature with preserved mental clarity is a diagnostic feature of the condition, "The patient retains his intelligence."[52] Poncet describes the classical form of this facial distortion, the sardonic smile, the *rire sardonique* (365), but adds that the distortion of the face by muscle spasm may be so severe that a physician may have difficulty recognizing a patient after its cure, "the natural expression of the face is absolutely changed and assumes a quality such that a physician, not having known the patient before [the attack of] tetanus would not recognize him after recovery."[53] Galdós's description does not include the pain of the muscle spasms that are typical of tetanus, but the remainder of his clinical portrait surely belongs to this condition.

As far as the convulsions of mourning bystanders are concerned, difficulty was experienced at that time in distinguishing a true *grand mal* seizure from attacks of hysteria.[54] Torquemada's response to his son's death is one of foaming at the mouth, violent contractions of the limbs followed by profound stupor, all typical of a *grand mal* seizure. In contrast, Leré's attack is described much more briefly with stiffening of the limbs, lack of speech and a twisted face. Given the beliefs of the time and Leré's gender, it is likely that her fit would have been interpreted as hysterical. What links both, however, is their onset as a result of overpowering emotional stress, a cause identified in contemporary medical texts.

These episodes illustrate Galdós's knowledge of the detailed clinical picture and progress of a number of diseases of childhood. In addition, they

51 "La temperature atteint les plus hauts dégres connus, 42°, 43°" (367).

52 "Le malade conserve son intelligence" (421).

53 "l'expression naturelle du visage est absolument changée et prend un caractère tel qu'un médecin ne connaissant pas le malade avant le tetanus no le reconnaîtrait pas après la guérison" (366). This is an interesting observation in view of the fact that, in the absence of modern treatment, tetanus is almost uniformly fatal.

54 *Grand mal* (French "Great Sickness"): a convulsion associated with loss of consciousness.

reveal his fascination for the processes of dying, not only in the children described here but also in adults, such as Pepe Carrillo in *Lo prohibido*, and Mauricia la Dura and Fortunata in *Fortunata y Jacinta*. In fact, one might add, Galdós's descriptions are so graphic that many of them can be regarded as truly clinical.

In contrast with these detailed depictions, however, there are instances when a whole world of contemporary medicine is implied so fleetingly that the context is easily missed. Such occurs in *Fortunata y Jacinta* when we are given the background of the deformed and charmless Maximiliano Rubín. When Galdós says of Maxi's birth, "he was born at seven months and then fed with a bottle and by a goat,"[55] he refers to the field of premature infant care that was emerging in France in the 1880s. At that time, the survival of a premature infant of seven months' gestation weighing about 1200 grams (about 38% of the weight of a healthy baby born at full-term) had been uncommon. Statistics were difficult to compile since the majority of children were delivered at home. Furthermore, figures derived from public institutions tend to represent infants of the sick and the poor, and infants submitted to last-ditch transfer, in a state that was often precarious. With these factors in mind, a review of the survival of infants weighing less than 2000 grams at the *Maternité de Cochin* and the *Maternité de Paris* in 1883 indicated a mortality of 66%. Though the nature of infant prematurity, *faiblesse congénitale*, was incompletely understood, Stéphane Tarnier (1828–97) achieved significantly improved rates of survival in 1881 when he improvised the first infant incubators, *couveuses*, which were warmed with tanks of heated water.[56] News such as this from a major Paris institution must have come to the attention of Tolosa Latour, who attended a conference there in 1883. Upon his return he would, no doubt, have been

55 "había nacido de siete meses y luego se le criaron con biberón y con una cabra" (*Fortunata I* 459–50).

56 Auvard reports an annual mortality of infants under 2000 grams in two maternity units in Paris of 65–66%, a rate comparable to the mortality of all infants, both premature and at term, seen in foundlings' hospitals in Madrid. After introduction of the *couveuse* (incubator) at the hospital of *Maternité*, the mortality was almost halved (38%) (1025–26).

ready to share the information with his novelist friend. A surviving seven-month gestation infant, a *sietemesino* such as Maximiliano, would have been of some topical interest in 1886, though no incubator would have been available in the 1850s for the fictional Maximiliano, the period that Galdós gives us for his birth.

An additional factor prejudicing the survival of premature infants was spoilage of the milk with which they were fed.[57] For although Pasteur had developed the technique of controlled heating followed by rapid cooling (pasteurization) in order to prevent spoilage of wine and beer as early as 1862, the process was not immediately applied to milk. It was not until 1886 that Ritter von Soxhlet successfully pasturized milk to make it safe for infant consumption (Rosenau 187). What made the problem worse was the dilution and adulteration of milk that were all but universal in big cities.[58] The mortality of even full-term infants fed spoiled milk from unwashed bottles in a foundlings' hospital like the Madrid institution of *La Inclusa* could reach 85%, leading to Tolosa Latour's well-deserved warning that, "to tolerate the feeding bottle is to condone infanticide."[59] The death rate at foundlings' hospitals led Concepción Arenal to observe that, "the

57 Brochard's struggle to draw attention to the excessive mortality of new-born infants in France in the 1870s is described by Routh (57 ff.). Routh quotes Becquerel and Vernois' study of adulteration of milk in Paris before documenting similar practice in English cities (312).

58 This is frequently mentioned in contemporary texts. A classic description of adulteration of milk and many other foods in Madrid is that of Serrano Fatigati in 1883. Routh (1876) records outbreaks of typhoid fever in England due to contaminated water being used to dilute milk or wash out milk containers (314–15). Even after pasteurization of milk was introduced in 1886, high infant mortality due to enteric diseases in France remained a national problem and only began to decline in the late 1890s (Budin 5–6). Rosenau emphasizes the inevitable separation of milk producer from consumer accompanying the growth of big cities, leading to a greatly increased delivery time of up to 48 hours (7–8, 258–60). There was no safe refrigeration at the time.

59 "tolerar el biberón es absolver el infanticidio" (*Niño* 88, 71) Similar conditions in hospitals in Paris at the time are described by Rachel Fuchs (137–38).

foundlings now die at such a rate that if the survival of the species were to rely upon them alone, it would become extinct."[60]

The Paris paediatrician, Joseph Parrot (1829–1883), encountered many infants with congenital syphilis that had traditionally been suckled by wet-nurses. However, this practice ran the risk of infecting the nurses, who then passed the contagion to other infants they suckled in the nursery, and to their own families. Such hazards were well-recognized and gave rise to medico-legal and social problems that occurred when wet-nurses concealed their infection from their employers, or vice versa. Tolosa Latour was aware of the problem in Spain for he describes the tragedy of a young man who, knowing himself to be infected, marries and passes on his disease to his unwitting wife and to their children. He mentions the lawsuits brought by wet-nurses and their families against parents who conceal their infection, citing the writings of Diday and Fournier in France.[61]

Tackling the problem of transmission of the disease in hospitals, Parrot adopted the traditional, rural custom, advocated by Boudard in 1876, of having syphilitic infants suckled directly by a donkey or a goat (*Nourricerie* 852). This practice relied on the fact that the nursing animals, being species that were not susceptible to human syphilis, could not acquire the infection from humans nor transmit it to them. Parrot studied the results of animal lactation on infant survival and also examined the nutritional value of the milk of the cow, the donkey and the goat. In a resulting series of 86 syphilitic infants in the foundlings' *Hospice des Enfants Assistés*, the results were sufficiently favourable for him to be able to proclaim that, "in the absence of a good wet-nurse, direct suckling directly from the teat of animals can be very useful. It is positively indicated for infant suffering from congenital syphilis."[62] For its value in avoiding unsafe milk in a bottle, and

60 "Los expósitos mueren ahora en una proporción tal, si á ellos solos estuviese confiada la conservación de la especie, se extinguiría" (*Cartas* 341).

61 Tolosa Latour, *Protección* 19–21. The problem was the subject of a long article published in 1877 in installments by Fournier (*Nourrices*).

62 "A défaut d'une bonne nourrice, l'allaitement direct au pis des animaux peut rendre de grands services. Il est formellement indiqué pour les enfants atteints de syphilis héréditaire" (*Nourricerie* 852).

for eliminating the transmission of syphilis, animal lactation was widely practised in France and was similarly recommended in Spain by Tolosa Latour (*Niño* 68, 72–73), Monlau (*Higiene* 523–24) and Viñeta-Bellaserra (*Profilaxia*), and in England, by Routh (443).

The Catalán syphilologist Viñeta-Bellaserra was very familiar with this technique of avoiding the infection of wet-nurses. However, he does caution, based on the contemporary belief in the role of suckled milk in the inheritance of personality (lactational heredity), that care should be taken that infants do not acquire the more undesirable personality traits of the goat:

> An infant suckled by goats involves the disadvantage of transmitting by absorption [of its milk] the disturbing events to which the animal is subject, exercising a harmful effect upon the weak infant's temperament, making it impatient and nervous [...] the *Asistencia Pública* of Paris, following professional advice, substituted goats with donkeys.[63]

He counsels that infants are better off if they acquire by ingestion the more socially desirable personality traits of the donkey.

Contemporary reviews of Galdós's novels appear to pay scant attention to their heart-wrenching depictions of childhood demise. It might, perhaps, be argued that high child mortality was so very much a part of everyday life in Madrid at the time that literary critics did not consider it worthy of special mention. If so, this would contrast with Tolosa Latour's medical text, *El Niño*, where he quotes the death of Monina from croup in *León Roch* as an authentic picture of, "croup, the greatest of all those monsters, as related by a talented observer who portrays admirably a night

63 "Un niño amamantado por una cabra [...] ofrece el inconveniente de comunicar por su absorción los accidentes nerviosos á que está sujeto el animal, ejerciendo una influencia maléfica sobre el temperamento del niño débil, poniéndole impaciente y nervioso [...] la *Asistencia Pública* de París, siguiendo los consejos facultativos, sustituyó las cabras por burras" (*Profilaxia* 27, author's italics).

of unbounded anguish such as those frequently endured by many doctors, but which are described truly by very few novelists."[64]

Even before being exposed to the often mortal infectious diseases of childhood, a potentially perilous phase through which newborn infants of Galdós's time had to pass was that of breast feeding. Galdós engages in this topic light-heartedly in *El amigo Manso* where the central charcter, Máximo, finds himself under pressure to secure the services of a wet-nurse for a godson at short notice. The official policy of the medical profession since the eighteenth century had been that breast-feeding should be undertaken by the infant's own mother whenever possible. Exceptions were recognized, such as when the mother's supply of milk was insufficient, or her health was considered to be too delicate to breastfeed. These considerations were modified in practice, however, by powerful social forces that emanated from the example of the royal family where the employment of wet-nurses was a longstanding tradition.[65] The nobility and the socially-conscious middle class tended to follow this royal example. In addition, there was an erroneous belief that marital relations would impair the quality of the mother's milk. Husbands unwilling abstain from conjugal sexual intercourse for a period that might last for years favoured engagement of a wet nurse so that their wives could suppress their lactation and become

64 "crup, el mayor de todos los monstruos como dice un observador de talento al pintar admirablemente una noche de angustias infinitas como las que pasan con frecuencia muchos médicos, y describen con verdad muy pocos novelistas" (*Niño* 188). As already mentioned the editor of *La hygiene*, Benito Áviles, also remarked on the authenticity of Galdós's depiction of diphtheria.

65 An ostensible justification for this practice was that the queen or consort should be liberated from the demands of suckling her children so that she could attend to her royal duties. It has been suggested that a secondary motive may have been that as lactation suppressed fertility and the monarch's duty was to provide as many heirs as possible to guarantee the survival of the dynasty, the queen/consort's priority was to become fertile as soon as possible after producing a child. This meant curtailing her lactation in favour of a wet nurse. Junceda Avello writes that suckling of a child by her mother at court, "was poorly regarded by the wives of courtiers and by royal couples, obsessed with the succession," "estaba mal visto entre las courtesanas y en los matrimonios reales, obsesionadas por la sucesión" (25–27).

sexually available again.[66] In addition to these consideratons, breast feeding tended to be regarded as a burdensome and menial occupation that was to be avoided by all who could afford to do so (Espinilla 69). Consequently, medical opinion was widely ignored and an industry involving large numbers of nursing mothers for hire developed to cater for the demands of the wealthy, and those who wished to imitate them. A consequence of this was that the public appearance of a well-nourished infant accompanied by an elegantly dressed wet-nurse became a desirable public ostentation, reflecting favourably upon the wealth and social position of the parents.[67]

Although the demand for wet-nurses was gradually diminishing in the last third of the nineteenth century,[68] the medical profession found itself obliged to vet the health of women who offered their services in Spain's major cities. Among the candidates for the position of wet-nurse, or *ama de cría*, were not a few prostitutes some of whom suffered from a variety of venereal diseases, the most feared of which was syphilis. It was well-recognized that wet-nurses could infect a suckling infant, and that the disease could be communicated to the mother, and hence to the entire family. Attempts to lessen this danger revolved about two measures. The first was to hire wet-nurses from agricultural areas associated with good health and freedom from the evils of urban prostitution. The second was the *reconocimiento*, a mandated medical examination, in which the general health of the candidate was assessed and the quality of her breast milk assayed. The examination included a search for any of the skin rashes or eruptions associated with secondary syphilitic disease, and examination of the internal genital tract

66 "Even husbands were in favour of this habit [of their wives' suppressing lactation in favour of a wet-nurse], believing as they did that it was unhealthy to have sexual relations during lactation," "Incluso los mismos maridos se mostraban partidarios de tal tendencia, creyendo como creían, que era perjudicial para la salud el mantener relaciones sexuales durante las lactancia" (Junceda Avello 27).

67 "The wet-nurse in a home soon came to be seen as a sign of the social position of the family [...] an indispensable part of the image of the wealthy classes," "La nodriza en casa pasó pronto a ser vista como un signo del la posición social de la familia [...] elemento indispensable de la imagen de las clases opulentas" (Sarasúa 180, 183).

68 Del Amo Del Amo 563.

for signs of venereal sores, as it was clear to the medical authorities of the 1870s that the traditional *ad hoc* arrangements were too open to abuse.[69] So when Galdós jocularly refers to, "the all encompassing vigilance of our administration," *la vigilancia omnímoda de nuestra administración* (323) he is, in fact, referring to the government response to the very real hazards of disease that could be spread by suckling from unhealthy wet-nurses. Augusto Miquis' work in the *Gobierno Civil* would have been mandated by the "Regulation for the inspection of public health in the sections of hygiene of wet-nurses and prostitutes," which was introduced in 1877 and which stipulated the medical supervision of women entering the market.[70] When Galdós describes the harried Manso casting about to find a suitable wet-nurse for his newborn godson, he includes much detail of the social and medical customs surrounding the wet-nurse industry prevalent in 1879–81, the period in which the action of *Amigo Manso* transpires.

Since the 1830s the traditional place in Madrid for marketing the services of these wet-nurses was the plazuela de Santa Cruz.[71] The most sought-after of these *amas de cría* came from the the *cornisa cantábrica*, the

69 A very detailed guide to the thorough examination of the prospective wet-nurse is that of López Arrójo. It is full of references to the lesions produced by syphilis that had to be sought.

70 *Reglamento de la Inspección de Salubridad Pública en sus secciones de higiene de las nodrizas y de la prostitución*. In recommending centres for the medical examination of wet-nurse, Tolosa Latour refers to it in *El niño*, "An office of this type has already been established in Madrid" "Ya en Madrid hay establecida una dependencia de este género" (74) The title of the *Reglamento* implicitly recognizes the possibility of overlap of the two occupations.

71 Mesonero Romanos describes the Plaza de Santa Cruz and its market of wet-nurses in 1837. The women were typically drawn from the region of Santander for the reputed health and vigour of country women bred there (346–47). They became fashionable after María Cristina, Fernando VII's fourth consort, selected her wet-nurse from the area in 1831 (Sarasúa 183). Originally from the valleys of the rivers *Miera, Pisueña* and *Pas* in Cantabria, they acquired the name *pasiegas* and the term came to extend to all wet-nurses from the north of Spain. Galdós refers to wet-nurses in *Amigo Manso* as, "those many sent to us from the outlawed Pasiego mountains," "cuantas nos envían montes encartados y pasiegos" (320). A description of *pasiegas* in 1851 is also to be found in the poem-essay *La nodriza* of Bretón de los Herreros (570–71).

agricultural districts adjacent to the north coast. This market was supplemented by notices in the *Diario de Avisos* in which the number of women advertising their services varied between 1,135 and 1,924 a year between 1858 and 1868, representing over 80% of all advertisements for domestic service (Sarasúa 147). Physicians like Monlau warned of the importance of having a physician examine prospective wet-nurse to ensure that they were not suffering from diseases that could be communicated to the infant and the infant's family.[72] Monlau recommends the selection of married wet-nurses of medium physique, under 35 years of age, and who have been lactating for 4–6 months, preferably with experience of the care of infants after the delivery of at least a second child. Monlau recommends analysis of the candidate's breast milk for its cream content with the *lactoscope* devised by Donné, and advises that they should be well-fed, not be given alcohol, and have good teeth (519–20).[73]

In Galdós's novel, Manso first receives from his neighbour, doña Javiera, a likely source of wet-nurses at an establishment in the centre of Madrid, "Don't neglect to go to Matías' place on Concepción Jerónima where all the milk-mules will collect to look for [employment] as wet-nurses."[74] She then recommends that he consults newspaper advertisements. Only finally does she suggest that he attend the government facility where wet-nurses are examined, warning him that he needs to employ the services of a doctor and to choose a nurse with good teeth whose milk he has examined: "Go quickly to the Civil Government where the examination takes place. If

72 In recommending the need for examination of the genital tract of wet-nurse before they are employed, Monlau urges, "the safety of the parents and the children demands this [...] contagious infectious diseases will enter the heart of the purest families through the gateway of [mercenary] lactation," "así lo exigen la seguridad de los padres y la salud del hijo [...] las enfermedades contagiosas penetrarán en el seno de las familias más puras por el portillo de la lactancia" (*Higiene* 517).

73 The nineteenth-century controversy over the accuracy of Donné's qualitative analysis of breast milk in comparison with more laborious chemical analysis is discussed by Garrigós, Millán and Blanes.

74 "No deje usted de ir a la Concepción Jerónima, a casa de Matías, donde van a parar todas las burras de leche que vienen a buscar cría" (Benito Pérez Galdós. *El amigo Manso*. Ed. Francisco Caudet. Madrid: Cátedra, 2001. 321, hereafter cited as *Manso*).

you find one, don't trust appearances; engage a doctor. Choose one who is rough, mannish and ugly ... Large black breasts. Look out for the pretty ones, who are usually the worst ... Don't forget to look at the milk and pay attention to good teeth."[75]

Manso repairs immediately to the *Gobierno Civil* where he encounters his friend, the recurring Galdósian doctor Augusto Miquis, labouring to examine a large number of wet-nurses for hire, *el escuadrón mamífico* (*Manso* 323). Manso sees breasts palpated to determine whether their bulk is made up of muscle or fat (324), the latter being a better harbinger of milk secretion. The candidates have their teeth examined. Galdós then has Miquis, "look for signs of past mischief [heresy]," *rebuscar vestigios de pasadas herejías* (324). The expression suggests a *double entendre* on Galdós's part. On the one hand it tells us that Miquis is looking for tell-tale scars of previous venereal infection. On the other, it may be a reflection of the belief, widespread in the nineteenth century and already alluded to, in lactational heredity. It was believed that the temperamental, moral and personal qualities of a wet nurse could be transmitted to the infant as traits that could be life-long. Such beliefs had long been elaborated further to include the wet-nurse's religious persusion, such that she should be known to be Christian and of Christian antecedants in order that she not transmit religious heresies to the child.[76] In addition, a contemporary text on

75 "Váyase pronto al Gobierno Civil donde está el reconocimiento ... Si encuentra usted alguna, no se fíe de apariencias: llévese un médico. Escójala cerril, fea y hombruna ... Pechos negros y largos. Mucho cuidado con las bonitas, que suelen ser las peores ... No dejen de examinar la leche, y fíjense en la buena dentadura" (*Manso* 321–22). The ugly, manly and black-breasted features are not found in the texts I have examined and suggest satirical intent on Galdós's part, consistent with the rest of his jocular account of the *escuadrón mamífico*.

76 One of the advantages of wet-nurses from rural communities of Cantabria was considered to be that they were less likely to have their blood mixed with that of Moorish or Jewish antecedents, "less mixture of unchristian blood," "menor mezcla de sangres no cristianas" (Sarasúa 158). Junceda Avello observes, "It was accepted as highly likely that [breast] milk transmitted moral qualities, manners, beliefs, etc., and even that by this means heresy was spread, in a nation like ours in which Jews and converted Moors lived, more or less concealed," "Admitían como verosímil que

choosing a wet-nurse advises that she should have some native intelligence to pass on to the infant, "in the same way it is appropriate that she should have some [mental] ability [...] it is indubitable that she exercises a certain influence on the constitution and function of the [infant's] brain."[77]

Miquis then uses the lactoscope, *lactoscopio*, in order to examine a specimen of breast milk for its cream content. This is likely to be a reference to the instrument devised by Alfred Donné in 1843 that contained parallel glass plates between which the milk to be examined was introduced.[78] The instrument was then held up to a source of light, such as a candle, to assess it opacity and, hence, its fat content. Galdós describes Miquis performing exactly this manoeuvre as he holds the instrument containing its thin film of milk, against the light coming in from a window. Voelcker in 1863 describes the instrument in an English journal and comments that it, "does not give accurate results, and for this reason has never come into practical use" (315). Galdós may have been aware of its limitations for he has Miquis check his preliminary results with an instrument capable of more precise chemical analysis of milk fat, the *lacto-butirómetro*, "because there are counterfeits, my friend," *porque hay falsificaciones, amigo* (*Manso* 325).[79]

---

la leche transmitiese cualidades morales, costumbres, creencias, etc., y hasta incluso que por este medio se propagase la herejía, en un pueblo como el nuestro en el que vivían judíos y moriscos más o menos encubiertos" (27).

77 "Conviene asimismo que se halle adornada de cierta capacidad [...] es indudable que ejerce cierta influencia en la constitución y manera de funcionar del encéfalo" (Martínez y Suárez 81).

78 Garrigós Oltra et al 667.

79 The lactobutyrometer was extremely important in detecting the dilution of milk with water, a widespread form of adulteration of milk in cities in the nineteenth century. The best known device, which measured the amount of cream in milk chemically, was devised by Gerber in 1892, after *Amigo Manso* was written. An earlier instrument was invented by Eugène Marchand in 1855, and may have been the one that Galdós had in mind. Its use involved mixing measured quantities of caustic soda, ether and alcohol with a specimen of milk. The fat in milk was first dissolved by the ether and then precipitated by alcohol. The tube was then warmed in a water bath, when the fatty cream melts and forms a layer that enables its quantity to be measured. Voelcker observes that the instrument, "requires much dexterity on the part of the operator, and therefore is not likely to be used by persons who have no experience in chemical

At Manso's increasingly desperate urging, Miquis provides him with a one-eared wet-nurse from Segovia, "the only cow who is worth anything," *la única res que vale algo* (325). Crucially, he assures, Manso, that he can find in her no signs of infectious disease, *no hay señales de mal infeccioso* (326). As he leads her to his godson's household, Manso finds that she is accompanied by her father, her mother and two brothers, all strangely attired, unwashed and smelly. On arrival, the hungry Maximín takes well to the wet-nurse's breast, causing his mother such relief that she is happy to provide food and shelter for the accompanying tribe.[80]

Though brief, this episode in *Amigo Manso* again illustrates Galdós's unusual talent for researching medical details and introducing many of them, almost incidentally, to give authenticity to to his portrayal of an everyday scene in Madrid.

---

manipulation. In the hands of a professional chemist this instrument furnishes tolerably accurate results" (315). Donné's *lactóscopo* and Marchand's *lacto-butirómetro* are also described in López Arrójo's *Reconocimiento* (23–25).

80 This extreme example of the wet nurse's entire family being hosted by the infant's family is clearly intended to be humorous. In real life, Sarasúa finds, that it was uncommon for a wet-nurse to be able to care for even her own infant in her employer's home, "references to wet-nurses who had their [own] infants with them in the home where they worked are very few," "las referencias a nodrizas que tienen a sus hijos consigo en la casa donde trabajan son muy escasas" (163).

CHAPTER 8

Conclusions

The passages studied reveal an exceptional knowledge of medicine for a novelist. Galdós's use of medical detail is judicious, however, such that in the case of many sick characters of the novels their medical background is touched on lightly. As examples, the causes of the blindness of Manolo Trujillo in *Lo prohibido*, and Rafael de Águila in the *Torquemada* novels are not given. No doubt they are incidental to the metaphorical blindness that each displays in misinterpreting their differing life circumstances. The brief references to the cause of blindness of Lucía in *Ángel Guerra* (smallpox) and Almudena in *Misericordia* (infected water) are entirely secondary to the importance of their roles in the novels. In this they contrast with the blindness of Pablo Penáguilas in *Marianela* and Francisco Bringas in *La de Bringas* where details of the characters' loss of sight are central to the stories.

The majority of medical conditions portrayed by Galdós appear to have a wide social impact. In contrast with the personal and unshared illnesses of doña Lupe's mastectomy in *Fortunata y Jacinta* and the heroine's leg tumour that requires amputation in *Tristana*, the condition of most sick patients in Galdós has a palpable effect on the circle surrounding them. The visionary lunacy of Tomás Rufete, directly or indirectly, pervades all of *La desheredada*. Alejandro Miquis's slow demise is attended by a chorus of characters, many of them bent on taking advantage of him in his penury. Maximiliano Rubín's profound mental disturbance wreaks havoc upon the lives of those about him, while the tragic death of Ción serves to propel Ángel on his fatal path of false mysticism, and Leré toward her extreme ascetic ideal. Galdós seems to be telling us that disease is not a solitary experience but that it has powerful and unpredictable consequences for those who surround the sufferer. His studies of cholera and diphtheria, especially, must have made him aware that in respect of disease, *No man is an island, entire of it self.*

Galdos's idealization of the medical profession has been widely observed, especially as it revolves about his characters of Augusto Miquis, Moreno Rubio and Teodoro Golfín.[1] In this context, it is tempting to return to Galdos's prologue to Tolosa's *Niñerías* in which he likens his adoration of medicine, *la noble ciencia*, to that of a distant and unrequited lover, "a silent and resigned passion like those Platonic and unequal relationships in which the suitor passes his life looking from afar at his would-be betrothed [...] but not daring to offer himself in marriage."[2] It may be that this metaphor contains more truth than the author intended, since it can be easier to adore a distant and idealised beloved than to accommodate oneself to intimate, day-to-day contact with a person of flesh and blood. Life for the majority of doctors in Galdós's time, according to Marañón, Baroja and the contemporary medical press, was harsh, competitive, exhausting and often poorly rewarded. The most successful of Madrid's practitioners may have been able to live in an atmosphere of wide respect, and even adulation; Galdós's principal doctors are portrayed as belonging to this echelon. For the majority of those relegated to the lower middle class, however, professional life appears to have been a poorly regarded struggle both in cities and in the rural *partido*.

Characters of Madrid's lower middle class and lower classes tend to predominate in Galdós's novels, reflecting his preference for people from these backgrounds. He habitually chose to take his railway journeys in third-class carriages in the company of common folk, whose conversation and ways he studied.[3] When visiting Toledo, according to Marañón, he tended

1 A specific study is that of Willey.

2 "pasion silenciosa, resignada, como esos noviazgos platónicos y desiguales en que el galán se pasa la vida mirando de lejos á la que cree novia [...] mas sin atreverse á pretenderla en matrimonio" (*Prólogo* ii).

3 "I travel in third class, with no [additional] amenities in contact with simple and humble folk, enduring the discomforts of bad accommodation. I listen, observe and make notes mentally or sometimes on paper. Amongst those rustics I learn much," "Viajo en tercera, sin ninguna comodidad en contacto con gentes humildes y sencillas,

to spend his time in the company of unpretentious working people, and steered clear of officials and of those with titles.[4] Despite this, there seems to be no record of friendships with run-of-the-mill or struggling doctors, and he appears not to have included them in his fictional portraits. They thus appear to represent an exception to the plan of his original manifesto where he set out to portray the "middle-class" in all its strengths and weaknesses:

> The modern novel of daily life has to be the expression of whatever good and bad exists in the background of this [middle] class, of the unceasing agitation that it engages in, of that determination that it reveals to achieve certain ideals and resolve certain problems that concern everyone, and to recognize the origin and remedy of certain ills that trouble families.[5]

While Galdós reveals the "good and bad" aspects of the majority of his characters, doctors, seem to be spared this even-handed treatment. In *Marianela*, Teodoro Golfín's improbable rise to international eminence in his field from the humblest of circumstances is portrayed as the result of

---

sufriendo las molestias de malos alojamientos. Oigo, observo y apunto en la mente, alguna vez en papel. Entre esos rústicos aprendo mucho" (Morote).

4 "Galdós had very many friends in Toledo almost always from the social borderland between the working and the middle class, in which it gave him such pleasure to live [...] one never saw Galdós with officialdom [...] Nor did he take pleasure in aristocrats with dazzling titles, distinguished politicians nor any other class of society's high dignitories," "En Toledo tuvo Galdós numerosos amigos casi siempre de aquella capa social limítrofe entre el proletariado y la clase media, en la que le era tan grato convivir [...] jamás se vió a Galdós con personajes oficiales [...] Tampoco se hallaba a gusto con nobles de relumbrantes títulos, políticos de alto bordo ni ninguna otra clase de altos dignatarios de la sociedad" (*Elogio* 155–56). Elsewhere, Marañón writes, "[Galdós] always preferred the company of humble folk, above all characters of the common people, to that of complicated people," "[Galdós] prefirió siempre el trato de las gentes humildes, sobre todo el de los personajes del pueblo, al de los hombres complicados" (*Galdós* 27).

5 "La novela moderna de costumbres ha de ser la expresión de cuanto bueno y malo existe en el fondo de esa clase, de la incesante agitación que la elabora, de ese empeño que manifiesta por encontrar ciertos ideales y resolver ciertos problemas que preocupan a todos, y conocer el origen y el remedio de ciertos malos que turban las familias" (*Observaciones* 167).

single-mindedness and unalloyed determination (148–51). In *La desheredada* Augusto Miquis seems to ascend rather easily to the medical directorship of one of Madrid's principal hospitals (299). Augusto Miquis, Moreno Rubio and Golfín represent an ideal model to be admired and emulated, contrasting with the failings of other characters. The counterpoint in *La desheredada* between the professional ascent of Augusto Miquis, as a result of his solid bourgeois values, and the descent of Isidora, with her obsessive delusion of nobility, illustrates this eloquently. No doctor, however, is shown enduring the type of hard-scrabble struggle that Felipe Centeno and Ramón Villaamil experience, although we know that in real life in Madrid at that time it was the rule rather than the exception. When Galdós portrayed, "whatever good and bad exists in the background of this [middle] class," he chose to elide the manifold ills with which the medical middle classes had to contend.

It appears likely that Galdós represented doctors in this idealized manner not because of an unrepresentative impression given to him by his elite circle of medical friends but because they embodied the "certain ideals" to which he felt Spanish society should aspire. The values that he espoused himself: liberalism, hard work, concern for and kindness toward others, and receptivity to new ideas, especially those emanating from positivist science, are those that appear in his physicians.[6] Marañón's observation that physicans had an iconic significance for nineteenth-century liberals

6 Unamuno found Galdós's ideals ingenuous, "they were, perhaps, reducible to the generous and romantic belief in progress of [...] the Spanish revoution of 1868, though simple and naïve in the extreme," "se reducía acaso al progresismo generoso y romántico, pero cándido de sobra, sencillo, de [...] la Revolución española del año 1868" (1203). From the perspective of the 1950s, Granjel summarizes these liberal beliefs, "those professed by the convinced and adepts of liberal and anticlerical, nineteenth-century naturalism, coloured by humanitarianism and faith in an unlimited, utopian perfectibility of human nature," "los profesados por los convictos y confesos adeptos del naturalismo decimonónico, liberal y anticlerical, teñido de humanitarismo y fe en un utópico perfeccionamiento sin límites de la naturaleza humana" (*Médico* 175).

appears close to the mark; to be effective as icons their darker side had to be be suppressed.[7]

Such was his admiration for this "kind of noble fraternity both scientific and religious" (*Prólogo* iv), that at one point he declares himself likely to be upstaged by their profession in the search for the novelist's Holy Grail, an understanding the well-springs of human passions, "I am certain that if we were able to master [Medicine] and it were possible for us to reveal the secret of the temperaments and of functional disorders, the diagnosis of the passions would not be so mysterious and complex."[8]

Occasionally, Galdós's conflation of the physician as scientist and as an infinitely caring human being is an uncomfortable one. This is notably true in Augusto Miquis who, in his enthusiasm for clinical medicine, is able to see in a hospital full of suffering and dying patients, "a thousand varieties of threatened lives and a thousand types of death [...] infinite manners of suffering" feeding the "supreme good, Science."[9] We are invited to consider the beautiful flowers of science arising from the repugnant manure of suffering humanity, "the plant of beautiful and aromatic flowers is simply a transformation of the common and disgusting substances contained in the earth and in manure."[10] This apparent complacency in the face of so much suffering seems far removed from the experience of Madrid hospitals, as related by Baroja and Marañón. We may choose to attribute this discrepancy either to Miquis' callow enthusiasm as a youthful student, or perhaps, to Galdós's lack of experience of hospitals, apart from the asylum of Leganés.

7 "This prestige that the physicians had in the mind of the liberals of the nineteenth century was, to a certain extent, a preoccupation of the century" (*Elogio* 145).

8 "tengo la certidumbre de que si lográramos conquistarla [la Medicina] y nos revelara el secreto de los temperamentos y de los desórdenes funcionales, no sería tan misteriosa y enrevesado para nosotros el diagnóstico de las pasiones" (*Prólogo* viii).

9 "mil especies de vidas amenazadas y mil categorías de muertes [...] infinitos modos de sufrir" (*desheredada* 129).

10 "la planta de flores hermosas y aromáticas es simplemente una transformación de las sustancias vulgares o repugnantes contenidas en la tierra y en el estiércol" (*desheredada* 129).

This far-from-invariable combination of enthusiastic scientist and deeply caring clinician is part and parcel of Galdós's idealization of the profession.

To be sure Galdós provides less idealized depictions in a few of his secondary medical figures. Quevedo in the *Torquemada* novels is dominated by his disdainful father-in-law and ironically shares his name with the seventeenth century satirist who savagely criticised the medical profession.[11] Quevedo is almost reduced to tears when Augusto Miquis takes him to task for his incorrect diagnosis and mismanagement of Fidela's severe heart disease (529). In *Lo prohibido*, José María provides a tart assessment of the smooth-talking but ineffectual Zayas, who is called to treat Pepe Carrillo, "that doctor was no champion of science [...] If the mission of the doctor is to entertain the sick and to raise their spirits with ingenious words and even meatphors, Zayas was unequalled. For the rest, he never cured anyone, ever."[12] In the ranks of unnamed physicians in the novels, criticism becomes more frequent. It may be implied by circumstances, as in the asylum doctor of Leganés in *La desheredada*, who may be "serious and kind," *serio y bondadoso*, but this does not prevent him or a colleague from referring Tomás to the brutal cold showers that kill him. The first physician to treat Francisco Bringas turns out to be an bumbler who is out of his depth and who cannot even distinguish retinal disease at the back of the eye from conjunctivitis at the front. The cabal summoned to advise on the dying Fidela in *Torquemada y San Pedro* provides no help apart from confirming Augusto Miquis' diagnosis (534). In contrast, the unnamed *médico de la Beneficencia domiciliaria* who attends Mauricia la Dura in her last illness in *Fortunata* (*II* 171) appears to be quietly efficient and to know what he is doing, and the two physicians who treat Dulcenombre, one in Toledo and the other in Madrid, seem able to effect a cure of her incipient alcoholism without further comment.

11 Willey 94.

12 "El tal doctor no era una notabilidad de la ciencia, [...] Si la misión del facultativo es entretener a los enfermos y alegrar su espíritu con ingeniosas palabras y aun con metáforas, Zayas no tiene quien le eche el pie adelante. Por lo demás, ni él curaba a nadie, ni Cristo que lo fundó" (323).

Other unnamed physicians, who are the butt of some of Galdós's bitterest attacks, are the medical authorities charged with limiting the spread of cholera. In his press articles Galdós upbraids the anonymous medical collective for its endless theoretical wrangling and its inability to devise public health measures that would afford protection to the community. Galdós identified medical mediocrity and incompetence in the face of uncertainty in the profession about how cholera was transmitted.

What emerges from this study of Galdós's medical knowledge is not only its depth but also the author's awareness of recent medical discoveries. At a time when the connection between syphilis and G.P.I. had only recently been propounded and remained controversial, he portrays the association unequivocally in Maximiliano Rubín. His portrait of neurasthenia in José María Bueno de Guzmán was penned within a few years of its first description in book form. While choosing to disregard the patent impossibility of the miraculous restoration of Pablo Penáguilas' sight after cataract removal, he nevertheless inserts an easily missed reference to *capas corticales* that suggests that he was aware of recent work in the localization of visual function in the cerebral cortex. His assessment of the controversy over Ferrán's cholera vaccine, and the issues that it stimulated in the nascent field of immunology, reads very well in retrospect. Even allowing for his liberal sympathies, his layman's analysis of the Catalan's work is exemplary.

As a realist writer, Galdós creates an illusion that resonates with the reader's perception of real life. An indication of his success in creating that illusion is that, on occasion, it attains the quality of a social document. It is as such that the historian of the nineteenth century, Manuel Tuñon de Lara, cites the visit of Juanito Santa Cruz and his new bride to a textile mill in Cataluña and Jacinta's reactions to the harsh working conditions she sees there (*Fortunata* 25). He further praises the verisimilitude of Galdós's description of the wretched living conditions of Madrid's poor in, "A Visit to the fourth estate," *Una visita al cuarto estado* in chapter 9 of *Fortunata y Jacinta*.[13] A strong case can be made that Galdós's *novelas contemporáneas*

13 "'A visit to the fourth estate,' is an irreplaceable document for the knowledge of the conditions of workers' dwellings in Madrid of those times," "'Una visita al cuarto

contain not only social history but also documents of medical history. Diphtheria before the era of endotracheal intubation and antitoxin therapy, and tetanus at the time that its bacteriology was being established, but long before vaccination was developed, are depicted in the novels. As such they record an historical phase of medical practice that began to disappear in Western Europe by the end of the 1880s. In contrast, Galdós's portraits of terminal pulmonary tuberculosis and congenital syphilis leading to G.P.I., now fortunately rare in the Western world, remained topical well into the twentieth century. Galdós's depictions of disease retain their documentary veracity, in contrast with his portrayals of triumphant doctors, "*los triunfadores*" (Marañón, *Vocación* 336), who seem to escape the narrative of realism to occupy a sphere of more idealized fiction.

It is tempting to look at Galdós's background in an attempt to account for why he should have been so interested in medicine, and what purpose is served in his novels by his depictions of disease. The history of his childhood available to us is one of a timid and highly imaginative child, the last child of a domineering mother and an unassertive father, spoiled by his older sisters. There seems to be no history of unusual exposure to death or disease at this stage in his life. He was known among his peers for his sharply observed pencil portraits that verged on caricature, though without any preference for the pathological.

The role of diseased characters in his novels is less difficult. The Naturalist poetic of the novel derived from Zola and his contemporaries was committed to the depiction of aspects of life that previous realist writers found unpalatable. In his passion to understand the "secret of the temperaments and of functional disorders" of his characters, many of whom were based on people he knew, it seems likely that he found at least a partial explanation in recognized patterns of eccentricity and madness. This explanation must be incomplete, however, since madness appears in his very earliest stories, *La novela del tranvía* and *La sombra* that antedate

---

estado,' es un documento irremplazable para conocer las condiciones de la vivienda obrera en Madrid de aquellos tiempos" (26).

the advent of Naturalism in Spain.[14] As Galdós wanted to diagnose the "source of the passions" of his characters, he may have found in disease a narrative that made them less "mysterious and complex," though the ultimate source, of course, remains elusive. In the broad foundation of Galdós's work, his well-informed and vivid depictions of disease play a significant though underestimated aspect of his genius. It is hoped that this study will provide a point of departure for further investigation.

14 Pattison dates this to 1879–1880 (84 ff.).

Bibliography

Abadie, Charles. "Nystagmus." *Nouveau dictionnaire de médecine et de chirurgie pratiques* Vol. 24. Paris: Baillière et fils, 1877.

Ackerknecht, Erwin H. "Anticontagionism between 1821 and 1867." *Bulletin of the History of Medicine* 22 (1948): 562–93.

——. *A Short History of Psychiatry*. Trans. Sula Wolff. 2nd ed. New York: Hafner Publishing, 1968.

Alas, Leopoldo. "Clarín." *Benito Pérez Galdós: (Estudio Crítico Biográfico)*. Madrid: Fe, 1889.

——. *Galdós novelista*. Ed. Adolfo Sotelo Vázquez. Barcelona: Universitas-15 PPU, 1991. 7–26.

Albarracín Teulón, Agustín. "Intrusos, charlatanes, secretistas y curanderos. Aproximación sociológica al estudio de la asistencia médica extracientífica en la España del siglo XIX." *Asclepio* 24 (1972): 323–66.

——. "La profesión médica ante la sociedad española del siglo XIX." *Asclepio* 25 (1973): 303–16.

——. "La titulación médica en España durante el siglo XIX." *Cuadernos de historia de la medicina española* 12 (1973): 15–79.

Almirall, Valentí. *España tal como es*. (1887) Trans. Rosario Fernández-Cancela. pról. Antoni Jutglar. Madrid: Seminarios y Ediciones, S.A., 1972.

Althaus, Julius. "Professor Ray Lankester and the Cholera Bacillus." *Pall Mall Gazette* 9 Oct. 1884. 1–2.

Álvaro, L.C. y Á. Martín del Burgo. "Trastornos neurológicos en la obra narrativa de Benito Pérez Galdós." *Neurología* 22.5 (2007): 292–300.

"Año nuevo." *El siglo médico* 6 Jan. 1889: 2–4.

Arenal, Concepción. "Cartas a un obrero No. 26. De la familia-El género humano no puede existir sin ella." *Obras completas* Vol. 7. Madrid: Lib. Victoriano Suárez, 1895. 331–42.

——. "El pauperismo Vol. 1." *Obras completas* Vol. 15 Madrid: Lib. Victoriano Suárez, 1897.

Armangué y Tuset, José. *Estudios clínicos de neuropatología*. Barcelona: Est. Tip. Sucs. Ramírez y Cía., 1884.

——. *Mimicismo ó neurósis imitatante* (*miriachit, jumping, latah*). *Estudio crítico*. pról. Juan Giné y Partagas. Barcelona: Est. Tip. Sucs. Ramírez y Cía., 1884.

Auvard, A. "De la couveuse pour enfants." *L'Union Médicale* 15 Dec. 1883: 1025–29.

Avilés, Benito. Apéndice: "Higiene pública según sus aplicaciones en España." *Tratado de higiene pública según sus aplicaciones en diferentes países de Europa.* Alberto Palmberg. Trans. Benito Avilés. Madrid: Est. Tip. Enrique Teodoro, 1892. 701–945.

——. "Homenaje á Pérez Galdós." *La higiene* 28 Mar. 1882. 90–91.

Bandrés, Javier, Rafael Llavona and Javier Campos. "Luis Simarro." *Personajes para una historia de la psicología en España.* Ed. Milagros Saiz and Dolores Saiz. Madrid: Ediciones Pirámide, S.A., 1996. 185–99.

Barbón-García, J.J., M.L Álvarez-Suárez and L. Sánchez-Tabar. "La ceguera y otras enfermedades oculares en las novelas de Galdós, *I* and *II*." *Archivos de la Sociedad Española de Oftalmología* 80.9 (2005): 551–53; 80.10 (2005): 623–24.

Baroja, Pío. *El árbol de la ciencia.* Ed. Pío Caro Baroja. Madrid: Cátedra, 1990.

——. "El aristocratismo en España." "Rapsodias" (1936) *Obras Completas V.* Madrid: Biblioteca Nueva, 1948. 957–61.

——. "De estudiante." "Ensayos: Juventud, Egolatría." (1917) *Obras Completas V.* Madrid: Biblioteca Nueva, 1948. 196–99.

——. "De estudiante de medicina." "Familia, infancia y juventud." Quinta Parte (1944). *Obras Completas VII.* Madrid: Biblioteca Nueva, 1949. 571–61.

——. "De médico de pueblo." "Familia, infancia y juventud." Sexta Parte (1944) *Obras Completas VII.* Madrid: Biblioteca Nueva, 1949. 613–34.

——. *Desde la última vuelta del camino III.* Barcelona: Tusquets Editores S.A., 2006.

——. "Galería de tipos de la época." *Obras Completas VII.* (1947) Madrid: Biblioteca Nueva, 1949.

——. "Recuerdos de un médico de pueblo." "Ensayos Intermedios." (1931) *Obras Completas V.* Madrid: Biblioteca Nueva, 1948. 671–81.

Barrier, François-Marguerite. *Tratado practico de las enfermedades de los niños arreglado á las lecciones del Dr. D. Antonio Mayner.* Trans. Luis Oms y Garrigolas and José Orial Ferreras. Barcelona: Imp. Ramón Indar, 1843.

Barrios y Barrios, Pedro. "Un lamento de un rural." *El genio médico-quirúrgico* 7 May 1883: 213–14.

Beard, George M. *American Nervousness. Its Causes and Consequences. A Supplement to Nervous Exhaustion (Neurasthenia).* New York: G.P.Putnam, 1881.

——. "Neurasthenia, or Nervous Exhaustion." *The Boston Medical and Surgical Journal* 29 Apr. 1869: 217–21.

——. *A Practical Treatise on Nervous Exhaustion (Neurasthenia).* New York: William Wood and Co., 1880.

Becerro de Bengoa, Ricardo. "El Sacamantecas." *Revista de España* 24.136 (1891): 21–39, 146–70.

Bell, T.E. *Galdós and Darwin*. Woodbridge: Tamesis, 2006.

Bénichou, Claude. "Enquête et reflexions sur l'introduction des termes dégénérere(r), dégénération, dégénérescence dans les dictionnaires et encyclopédies scientifiques françaises a partir du $17^{\text{ème}}$ siècle." *Documents Pour l'Histoire du Vocabulaire Scientifique*. No. 5. Ed. Pierre Louis. Paris: Institut national de la Langue Française (C.N.R.S.), 1983.

Berkowitz, H. Chonon. *La biblioteca de Benito Pérez Galdós*. Las Palmas: Ediciones *El museo canario*, 1951.

——. *Pérez Galdós Spanish Liberal Crusader*. Madison: University of Wisconsin Press, 1948.

Boix Martínez, Raquel. "Enfermedad y sociedad en la obra de B. Pérez Galdós." Diss. Universidad Complutense de Madrid, 1994.

Bondeson, Jan. "Maternal Impressions." *A Cabinet of Medical Curiosities*. New York: W.W.Norton, 1997. 144–69.

Bornside, George H. "Jaime Ferrán and Preventive Inoculation Against Cholera." *Bulletin of the History of Medicine* 55 (1981): 516–32.

Bouchut, E., and Armand Deprés, eds. *Dictionnaire de medicine et de thérapeutique médicale et chirurgical*. 4th ed. Paris: Germar Baillière et $C^{\text{ie.}}$, 1883.

Boudard, A. *Guide pratique de la chèvre-nourrice au point de vue de l'allaitement des nouveaux-nés*. Paris: Libraire Germer Baillière, 1876.

Braun, Lucille V. "Galdós's Re-Creation of Ernestina Manuel de Villena as Guillermina Pacheco." *Hispanic Review* 38 (1970): 32–52.

Bravo Moreno, Fernando. *Síntomas de la patología mental que se hallan en las obras literarias de D Benito Pérez Galdós discurso leído en la sesión inaugural del curso de 1922–1923 en la Sociedad de Psiquiatría y Neurología*. Barcelona: Imprenta particular del Instituto Mental de la Santa Cruz, 1923.

Bretón de los Herreros, Manuel. "La nodriza." *Poesías*. Madrid: Imprenta Nacional, 1851. 566–75.

Breitmeyer, Bruno G. *Blindness: The Many Ways We Cannot See*. Oxford: Oxford University Press, 2010.

Budin, P. *Étude sur la mortalité de la première enfance*. (Rapport su une mémoire de MM. Balestre et Gilletta de Saint-Joseph de Nice). Melun: Imprimerie administrative, 1904.

Buffon, George-Louis Leclerc. "De la dégénération des Animaux." *L'Histoire Naturelle, générale et particulière, avec la description du Cabinet du Roi (1749–1767)*. Vol. 14. Paris: L'Imprimerie Royale, 1766. 311–74.

Buignet, H. "Atropine." *Nouveau dictionnaire de médecine et de chirurgie pratiques*. Vol. 4. Paris: Baillière et fils, 1866. 85–90.

Burke, John. "Angina Ludovici: A Translation together with a Biography of Wilhelm Frederick von Ludwig." *Bulletin of the History of Medicine* 7 (1939): 1115–26.

Bynum, William F. "Chronic Alcoholism in the First Half of the 19th Century." *Bulletin of the History of Medicine* 42.2 (1968): 160–85.

Cabezas García, Félix. *La medicina y los médicos en la obra de Pío Baroja*. Bilbao: Ediciones Beta III Milenio, S.L., 2012.

Calatraveño, Ldo./Dr. "Más sobre la cuestión del día." *El genio médico-quirúrgico* 30 Nov. 1881. 665–67.

Campos Marín, Ricardo. *Alcoholismo, medicina y sociedad en España (1876–1923)*. Madrid: Consejo Superior de Investigaciones Científicas, 1997.

——. "Criminalidad y locura en la Restauración. El proceso del cura Galeote (1886–1888)." *Frenia* 3.2 (2003): 111–45.

——. "Entre el vicio y la enfermedad: La construcción medicosocial del alcoholismo como patología en España (siglos XIX y XX)." *Trastornos Adictivos* 1.3 (1999): 280–86.

——, and Rafael Huertas García-Alejo. "El alcoholismo como enfermedad social en la España de la Restauración: problemas de definición." *Dynamis* 11 (1991): 263–86.

——. "Lombroso but not Lombrosians? Criminal anthropology in Spain." *The Cesare Lombroso Handbook*. Eds Paul Knepper and P.J. Yesehede. London: Routledge, 2013. 309–23.

Carceda, Lino. "Un temor justificado." *El siglo médico* 1 Feb 1874: 69–71; 22 Feb. 1874: 125–26.

Carlan, Decio. "Año nuevo-Proyecto de ley de instrucción pública-Apertura." *El siglo médico* 17 Jan. 1877: 1–4.

——. "Conferencia del Dr. Koch." *El siglo médico* 9 Nov. 1884: 705–08; 23 Nov. 1884: 739–42.

——. "Nombramientos-Certificaciones falsas." *El siglo médico* 14 Jan. 1877: 17–18.

——. "Revista de la semana." *El siglo médico* 4 Oct. 1974: 625–27.

—— ("C"). "La verdad acerca del gérmen del cólera de Koch por Ray Lankester." *El siglo médico* 8 Feb. 1885: 82–85.

Casalduero, J. *Vida y obra de Galdós (1843–1920)*. Madrid: Editorial Gredos, S.A., 1974.

Caudet, Francisco. "Introducción." Benito Pérez Galdós, *Marianela*. Madrid: Cátedra, 2003. 9–66.

"Causa de regicidio." *El liberal* 7 Feb. 1880: 4–5.

Cervera Barat, R. *Alcoholismo y civilización*. Valencia: Imp. de A. Cortés, Ballesteros, 1896.

Chadwick, Edwin. "Evidence before Select Committee (26 Jun. 1846)." *The Sessional Papers Printed by Order of the House of Lords* XXXII (1846): 106–20.

Chamberlin, Vernon. "The Blind and Other Physically Handicapped Characters in the Novels of Benito Pérez Galdós." Diss. University of Kansas, 1957.

Charcot, J.-M. "Un cas de suppression brusque et isolée de la visión mentale des signes et des objets, formes et couleurs." *Le Progrès Médical* 11 (1883): 568–71.

Cheselden, William. "An Account of some observations made by a young Gentleman, who was born blind, or lost his Sight so early that he had no Remembrance of ever having seen, and was couch'd between 13 and 14 Years of Age." *Philosophical Transactions* 35.402 (1728): 447–50.

Christie, Charles J. *Libro médico azul*. part 2. London: Burroughs Wellcome y C$^{ia.}$, 1884.

Comenge y Ferrer, Luis. *La medicina en el siglo XIX*. Barcelona: José Espasa, 1914.

"La conferencia del Dr. Esquerdo sobre Garayo (Saca-Mantecas)." [Revista de la Semana] *El genio médico-quirúrico* 31 Jan. 1881: 45–46.

Conseglieri, Ana, and Olga Villasante. "La imbecilidad como exención de responsabilidad: El peritaje de Esquerdo en el proceso judicial de Otero." *Frenia* 7 (2007): 213–28.

——. "Una regicida frustrado: La imbecilidad de Otero, según Esquerdo." *La gestión de la locura: conocimiento, prácticas y escenarios (España, siglos XIX–XX)*. Eds Juan Martínez Pérez, Juan Estévez, Merceses del Cura and Luís Víctor Blas. Cuenca: Ediciones de la Universidad de Castilla-La Mancha, 2008. 283–310.

Corbyn, Frederick. *A Treatise on the Epidemic Cholera as it has Prevailed in India*. Calcutta: Baptist Mission Press, 1832.

Cotard, J. "Folie." *Dictionnaire Encyclopédique des Sciences Médicales*. Vol. 3. Paris: G. Masson, 1879. 271–306.

Crissey, John T. and Lawrence C. Parish. *The Dermatology and Syphilology of the Nineteenth Century*. New York: Praeger Publishers, 1981.

Crosby, Alfred W. "The Early History of Syphilis: A Reappraisal." *American Anthropologist* 71.2 (1969): 218–27.

Darwin, Charles. *The Descent of Man*. (1874). Intro. H. James Birx. 2nd ed. New York: Prometheus Books, 1998.

——. *The Origin of Species* (1859). Foreword Patricia Horan. New York: Gramercy Books, 1979.

Darwin, Erasmus. *The Botanic Garden* (1791). Menston: The Scholar Press, 1973.

De la Nuez Caballero, Sebastián. *Biblioteca y archivo de la casa museo Pérez Galdós*. Madrid: Excmo. Cabildo Insular de Gran Canaria, 1990.

Dechambre, A. ed. *Dictionnaire encyclopédique des sciences médicales*. Vol. 17. Paris: G. Masson, 1882.

Del Amo del Amo, Mª Cruz. "La Familia y el trabajo femenino en España durante la segunda mitad del siglo XIX." Diss. U. Complutense, 2008.

Del Mazo, J. "Los manicomios de España." *El siglo médico* 30 Dec. 1888: 846–47.

Del Moral Ruiz, Carmen. *La sociedad madrileña fin de siglo y Baroja*. Madrid: Ediciones Turner, S.A., 1974.
Del Toro y Quartiellers, Cayetano. *Tratado de las enfermedades de los ojos y de sus accesorios*. 2 vols. Cádiz: Tip. La Mercantil, 1878.
Deval, Charles. *Traité théorique et pratique des maladies des yeux*. Paris: Lib.-Editeurs Charles Albessard et Bérard, 1862.
Dowbiggin, Ian R. *Inheriting Madness: Professionalization and Psychiatric Knowledge in Nineteenth-century France*. Berkeley: University of California Press, 1991.
Dujardin-Beaumetz, [Georges] and [R.H.I.] Audigé. *Recherches expérimentales sur la puissance toxique des alcools*. Paris: E. Donnard, 1878.
Durey, Michael. *The Return of the Plague: British society and the cholera 1831–32*. Dublin: Gill and Macmillan, 1979.
Eadie, M.J. "Sir Charles Locock and potassium bromide." *Journal of the Royal College of Physicians of Edinburgh* 42 (2012): 274–79.
Eleizegui, José de. *Don José María Esquerdo*. Madrid: Imp. Antonio Marzo, 1914.
Elliott, Leota W., and F.M. Kercheville. "Galdós and Abnormal Psychology." *Hispania* 23 (1940): 27–36.
Ellis, H.D., and M. Florence. "Bodamer's (1947) paper on prosopagnosia." *Cognitive Neuropsychology* 7 (1990): 81–105.
Eoff, Sherman H. *The Novels of Pérez Galdós. The Concept of Life as a Dynamic Process*. Saint Louis: Washington University Studies, 1954.
Escuder, José María. *Locos y anómalos*. Madrid: Est. Tip. Succ. De Rivadeneyra, 1895.
——. *Plus ultra*. Madrid: Est. Tip. G. Pedraza, 1890.
——. *Quemas y crímenes*. Valencia: Impr. de E. Pascual, 1881.
Espinilla Sanz, Beatriz. "La elección de las nodrizas en las clases altas, del siglo XVII al siglo XIX." *Matronas profesión* 14.3–4 (2013): 68–73.
Esquerdo, José María. "Conferencias sobre enfermedades mentales." *El anfiteatro anatómico español* 15 Apr. 1878: 77; 15 May 1878: 91–92; 22 May 1878: 103–04; 31 May 1978: 117; 30 Jun. 1878: 148–49; 15 Jul. 1878: 164–65; 31 Jul. 1878: 175–76; 15 Aug. 1878: 191–92; 31 Aug. 1878: 202–03; 15 Sep. 1878: 209–10.
——. *Locos que no lo parecen. Garayo el Sacamantecas*. Madrid: Imprenta del Hospicio, 1881.
Esquirol, Jean-Étienne Dominique. *Note sur la monomanie-homicide*. Paris: J.-B. Baillière, 1827.
Eyler, John M. *Victorian social medicine: the ideas and methods of William Farr*. Baltimore: Johns Hopkins University Press, 1979.
Falret, Jean-Pierre. *Des maladies mentales et des asiles d'aliénés*. Paris: J.-B.Baillière et Fils, 1864.
Farmacopea Oficial Española. 6th ed., Madrid: Tip. Gregorio Estrada, 1884.

Fatás y Montes, Luis. *La mortalidad de niños en Madrid. Causas y remedio*. Madrid: Est. Tip. De E. Teodoro, 1903.
Faus Sevilla, Pilar. "Epidemias y sociedad en la España del siglo XIX. El cólera de 1885 in Valencia y la vacunación Ferrán." José María López Piñero, Luís García Ballester and Pilar Faus Sevilla. *Medicina y sociedad en la España del siglo XIX*. Madrid: Sociedad de Estudios y Publicaciones, 1964. 287–399.
Féré, Charles. *La famille névropathique*. Paris: Ancienne Libraire Germer Ballière et Cie, 1898.
Fernández, Antonio. *Epidemias y sociedad en Madrid*. Barcelona: Editorial Vicens-Vives, 1985.
——. "Repercusiones sociales de las epidemias de cólera del siglo XIX." *V Congreso Nacional de la Sociedad española de historia de la medicina* Madrid: 29 Sep.–1 Oct. 1977: 127–45.
Fernández, Pura. *Eduardo López Bago y el naturalismo radical*. Amsterdam: Rodopi, 1995.
Fernández Sanz, Juan José. "1885: *El año de la vacunación Ferrán. Trasfondo político, médico, sociodemográfico y económico de una epidemia*." Madrid: Ramón Aceres, 1990.
Fishman, Ronald S. "Brain Wars: Passion and conflict in the localization of vision in the brain." *Documenta Ophthalmologica* 89 (1995): 173–84.
Fodéré, F.E. *Traite de médecine légale et d'hygiène ou police de santé*. 3 vols. Paris: L'Imprimerie de Mame, 1813.
Forbes, John, Alexander Tweedie and John Conolly, eds. *Cyclopedia of Practical Medicine*. Vol. 1. London: Sherwood, Gilbert, and Piper, and Baldwin and Craddock, 1833.
Forbes, R.J. *Short History of the Art of Distillation*. Leiden: E.J. Brill, 1948.
Fournier, Alfred J. *De l'ataxie locomotrice d'origine syphilitique*. Paris: G. Masson, 1882.
——. "Nourrices et nourrissons syphilitiques." *L'Union Medicale*. Paris: 1877: 733–37, 805–10, 865–67, 1013–19; 201–08, 318–22, 345–48, 453–58, 533–37, 581–85, 641–47, 729–31, 821–26.
——. *La syphilis du cerveau. Leçons cliniques recueillies par E. Brissard*. Paris: G. Masson, 1879.
——. *La syphilis héréditaire tardive*. Paris: G. Masson, 1886.
Foville, Achille. "Folie-étiologie." *Nouveau Dictionnaire de médecine et de chirurgie pratiques*. Vol. 15. Paris: J.-B.Baillière, 1872. 213–76.
——. "Kleptomanie." *Nouveau Dictionnaire de médecine et de chirurgie pratiques*. Vol. 19. Paris: J.-B.Baillière, 1874. 701–03.
Francos Rodríguez, José. *Patogenia de la sífilis: sus relaciones con algunas enfermedades crónicas*. Madrid: Imp. Enrique Teodoro, 1884.

Franz, Thomas R. "Galdós the Pharmacist: Drugs and the Samaniego Pharmacy in *Fortunata y Jacinta*." *Anales galdosianos* 22 (1987): 33–46.

Fuchs, Rachel G. *Abandoned Children: Foundlings and Children in Nineteenth-Century France*. Albany: State University of New York Press, 1984.

Fuentes Peris, Teresa. *Visions of Filth: Deviancy and Social Control in the Novels of Galdós*. Liverpool: Liverpool University Press, 2003.

García Almansa, Antonio. *Tracheotomía en el crup*. Cádiz: Imp. Rev. Med. Federico Joly, 1888.

García Lisbona, José Ramón. "Las ciencias médicas en la obra de Pérez Galdós." Diss. U. Zaragoza, 1992.

Garma, Ángel. "Jaqueca, pseudo-oligofrenia y delirio en un personaje de Pérez Galdós." *Ficción* 14–16 (1958): 84–102.

Garrido, Victoriano. *La cárcel o el manicomio. Estudio médico legal sobre la locura*. pról. José María Esquerdo. Madrid: Casa editorial de don José María Faquineto, 1888.

Garrigós Oltra, Lluís, Carlos Millán Verdú and Georgina Blanes Nadal. "Física *versus* tecnología química: un ejemplo de la polémica decimonónica alrededor de la precisión." *Actas VIII Congreso de la Sociedad Española de la Historia de las Ciencias y las Técnicas* (2004): 667–86.

Gelabert, Enrique. *De la prostitución, en sus relaciones con la Higiene, en el doble concepto de la profilaxis de la sífilis y de la reglamentación. Discurso leído en la sesión inaugural* [...] *en 14 de enero de 1886* [...] *Academia y Laboratorio de Ciencias Médicas de Cataluña*. Ramón Castejón Bolea. "Las enfermedades venéreas y la regulación de la sexualidad en la España contemporánea." *Asclepio* 56.2 (2004): 225.

Gelfand, Craig. "Diphtheria: Dr Joseph O'Dwyer and His Intubation Tubes." *Caduceus* 3.2 (1987): 1–34.

Genil-Perrin, Georges. *L'Idée de Dégénérescence en Medecine Mentale*. Paris: Alfred Leclerc, 1913.

Gijswijt-Hofstra, Marijke. "Introduction: Cultures of Neurasthenia from Beard to the First World War." Ed. Marijke Gijswijt-Hofstra and Roy Porter. *Cultures of Neurasthenia. From Beard to the First World War*. Amsterdam: Rodopi, 2001.

Giné y Partagas, Juan. *Tratado clínico iconográfico de las enfermedades venéreas y sifilíticas*. Barcelona: Tip. La Acad. Evaristo Ullastres, 1883.

——. *Tratado teórico-práctico de freno-patología ò estudio de las enfermedades mentales*. Madrid: Moya y Plaza, 1876.

Glick, Thomas F. "Science and the Revolution of 1868: Notes on the Reception of Darwinism in Spain." *La Revolución de 1868: Historia, Pensamiento, Literatura*. Ed. Clara E. Lida and Iris Zavala. New York: Las Américas Publishing Co., 1970. 267–72.

Goldman, Peter B. "Galdós' Pueblo. A Social and Religious History of the Urban Lower Classes in Madrid 1885–1898." Diss. Harvard University, 1971.

Goldstein, Jan. *Console and Classify: The French Psychiatric Profession in the Nineteenth Century*. Chicago: University of Chicago Press, 1987/2001.

Gómez Ferrer, Ramón. *La herencia orgánica considerada principalmente bajo el punto de vista de la higiene*. Diss. Universidad Central, 1884. (Ms. Ca 2538 (819) Biblioteca de Medicina, Universidad Complutense, Madrid), subsequently published in installments in *Crónica médica (Valencia)* (1884–85) volume 8.

Gordon, M. "The Medical Background to Galdós' *La desheredada*." *Anales galdosianos* 7 (1972): 67–77.

Goyanes, J. "San Martín y su obra: Conferencia dada en el Ateneo de Madrid en diciembre de 1920." *El siglo médico* (1925): 224–27, 251–53, 277–79.

Granjel, Luís S. "Francos Rodríguez y la medicina madrileña 'fin de siglo.'" *El ejercicio médico y otros capítulos de la medicina española*. Salamanca: Universidad de Salamanca, 1974. 205–18.

——. "Galdós y la medicina." *Baroja y Otras Figuras del 98*. Madrid: Ediciones Guadarrama, 1960. 251–59.

——. "El médico galdosiano." *Archivo Iberamericano de Historia de la Medicina y Antropología Médica* 6 (1954): 163–76.

Grasset, J. *Enfermedades del sistema nervioso*. 2 vols. Trans. M.E. Moré y Bargit, prol. Pedro Esquerdo y Esquerdo. Barcelona: Imp. Peninsular, 1880.

Guimón Ugartechea, José. "Los médicos en la obra de Pío Baroja." *Gaceta Médica del Norte* 17.2 (1967): 107–22.

Guislain, Joseph. *Lecciones orales sobre las frenopátias ó tratado téorico y práctico de las enfermedades mentales*. 2 vols. Trans. M. Carreras Sanchis and J. Torres Fabregat, 2nd ed. Madrid: Imp. Enrique Teodoro, 1881–82.

Gullón, Ricardo. *Galdós, novelista moderno*. Madrid: Editorial Gredos, S.A., 1966.

Gutiérrez Bueno, Pedro. *Instrucción práctica para destilar las aguas fuertes y otros espíritus ácidos*. Madrid: Blas Román, 1787.

Gutiérrez Jiménez, Federico. *Profilaxis de la tuberculosis*. Madrid: Imp. J. Aguado, 1875.

——. *Estudios medicosociales sobre la tuberculosis en la España de la Restauración*. Ed. Jorge Molero Mesa. Madrid: Ministerio de Sanidad y Consumo, 1987. 179–205.

Hammond, William. *Traité des maladies du système nerveux*. Trans. F. Labadie-Lagrave, Paris: J.-B. Ballière, 1879.

Hardy, Anne. *The Epidemic Streets: Infectious Disease and the Rise of Preventative Medicine 1856–1900*. Oxford: The Clarendon Press, 1993.

Harrison, Brian. *Drink and the Victorians: The Temperance Question in England 1815–1872*. London: Faber and Faber, 1971.

Hauser, Ph. *Estudios epidemiológicos relativos a la etiología y profilaxis del cólera. Basados en estadísticas, hechos y observaciones durante la epidemia.* 3 vols. Madrid: Imp. Fund. Manuel Tello, 1887.

——. "El cólera actual en España y sus enseñanzas para la historia." *Revista de España* 105 (1885): 389–420.

——. *Madrid bajo el punto de vista médico-social.* 2 vols. Madrid: Rivadeneyra, 1902. Ed. Carmen del Moral. 2 vols. Madrid: Editora Nacional, 1979.

——."El siglo XIX considerado bajo el punto de vista médico-social." *Revista de España* (1884): 202–24, 333–58.

Hernández Benito, Emiliano. *El oficio de oculista en España. Pasado y presente.* Salamanca: Real Academia de Medicina de Salamanca, 1975.

Herrera Hernández, Manuel. *Consideraciones sobre la ceguera de Benito Pérez Galdós.* Gran Canaria: Real Sociedad Económica de Amigos del País de Gran Canaria, 2006.

——. "Perspectivas de las cataratas de Benito Pérez Galdós." *Anales de la Real Academia Nacional de Medicina* 124.3 (2007): 495–509.

Herrera Rodríguez, Francisco. "Un cirujano y humanista singular: Alejandro San Martín y Satrústegui (1847–1908)." *Llull* 32.70 (2009): 386–96.

Hirtz, [ ]. "Belladone." *Nouveau dictionnaire de médecine et de chirurgie pratiques.* Vol. 4. Paris: Baillière et fils, 1866. 751–72.

Hodgson, Barbara. "Drink Me: Laudanum and Other Traditional Opiate Medicines." *In the Arms of Morpheus: The Tragic History of Laudanum, Morphine, and Patent Medicines.* Buffalo, New York: Firefly Books, 2001. 45–77.

Homolle, Georges. "Syphilis héréditaire," *Nouveau Dictionnaire de médecine et de chirurgie pratiques.* Vol. 34. Paris: J.-B.Baillière, 1883. 859–906.

Huertas, Rafael. "Madness and Degeneration, IV. The man of genius." *History of Psychiatry* 4 (1993): 301–319.

——. *Organizar y persuadir. Estrategias profesionales y retóricas de legitimación de la medicina mental española (1875–1936).* Madrid: Frenia S.C., 2002.

Huertas García-Alejo, Rafael. "Valentin Magnan y la teoría de la degeneración." *Revista de la Asociación Española de Neuropsiquiatría* 5.14 (1985): 361–67.

Hughlings Jackson, John. *Case of Large Cerebral Tumour without Optic Neuritits and with Left Hemiplegia and Imperception.* London: Harrison and Sons, 1876. (Also *Royal London Ophthalmic Hospital Reports* 8 (1876): 434).

Hutchinson, Jonathan. "On the Means of Recognizing the Subjects of Inherited Syphilis in Adult Life." *Medical Times and Gazette* 11 Sep. 1858: 264–65.

Iglesias, Yolanda. *Realismo científico en la obra de Benito Pérez Galdós: Un análisis de la función de los criterios de la psicología moderna.* Buenos Aires: Elaleph.com S.R.L., 2006.

Jaccoud, S. *Tratado de patología interna*. 3 vols. Trans. Joaquín Gassó and Pablo Leon y Luque. Ed. Francisco Santana y Villanueva. 4th ed. Madrid: Bailly-Bailliere, 1885.

James, William. *The Principles of Psychology*. 2 vols. London: Macmillan, 1891.

Jelly, F.A. "A Glance at Lunacy in Spain." *British Journal of Mental Science* 1 Jul. 1885: 193–98.

Jimeno Agiús, J. "El cólera en España durante el año 1885 part 1." *Revista de España* May – Jun. 1886: 497–514; "part 2." *Revista de España* Jul.–Aug. 1886: 5–36.

——. "Población de España part 1." *Revista de España* (1885): 333–68; "part 2." 551–91.

Jones, C.A. "Galdós's *Marianela* and the Approach to Reality." *Modern Language Review* 56.4 (1961): 515–19.

Junceda Avello. *Ginecología y vida íntima de las reinas de España*. 2 vols. Madrid: Ediciones Temas de Hoy, 1991/92.

Kaplan, Temma. "Positivism and Liberalism." *La Revolución de 1868. Historia, pensamiento, literatura*. Ed. Clara E. Lida and Iris M. Zavala pról. Vicente Llorens. New York: Las Américas Publishing Company, 1970. 154–66.

Kronik, John. "Galdós and the Grotesque." *Anales galdosianos Anejo* (1976): 39–54.

Laín Entralgo, Pedro. *La historia clínica. Historia y teoría del relato patográfico*. Madrid: Editorial Triascastela, 1998.

Lancereaux, Étienne. *De l'alcoolisme et de ses conséquences au point de vue de l'etat physique, intellectual et moral des populations*. Paris: E. Donnard, 1878.

Lannelongue, Odilon. "El rachitisme." *Nouveau Dictionnaire de Médecine et de Chirurgie Pratiques*. Vol. 30. Paris: Baillière et fils, 1881. 376–405.

Larsen, Kevin S. "Ido de Sagrario's Alimentary Madness." *Science, Literature and Film in the Hispanic World*. Ed. Jerry Hoeg and Kevin S. Larsen. New York: Palgrave MacMillan, 2006. 151–73.

——. "'El caso de Mauricia debe de examinarse detenidamente.' Aspectos médicos de un personaje de *Fortunata y Jacinta*." *La Torre. Revista de la Universidad de Puerto Rico* 3.10 (1998): 615–36.

——. "The Medical Background of *Fortunata y Jacinta*: The Case of Maxi's Migraines." *Ometeca* 3½-4 (1996): 410–38.

Lasègue, Charles and J. Falret. "La folie à deux." *Archives Générales de Médicine* 30 (1877): 257–97.

Latham, Dr. "On Symptoms-Auscultation." *The London Medical Gazette* 17.1 (1835–36): 426–32.

Legrain, Paul. *Dégénérescence social et alcoolisme*. Paris: Georges Carré, 1895.

Leyden, E. *Traité clinique des maladies de la moelle épinière*. Trans. Eugène Richard and Charles Viry. Paris: J.-B. Baillière et fils, 1879.

Linas, A. "Monomanie." in *Dictionnaire Encyclopédique des Sciences Médicales*. Vol. 9. Paris: G. Masson, 1875. 146–95.

Lloréns y Gallard, Ignacio. *La tuberculosis en Barcelona.* Barcelona: Est. Tip. Casa de P. Caridad, 1900.

Loeffler, F. "History of Diphtheria." *The Bacteriology of Diphtheria.* Ed. G.H.F. Nuttall and G.S. Graham-Smith. Cambridge: Cambridge University Press, 1908. 1–52.

López Arrójo, Lucio. *Reconocimiento de nodrizas.* 2nd ed. Madrid: Imp. M.P. Montoya, 1889.

López Piñero, José M. "La medicina y la enfermedad en la España de Galdós." *Cuadernos Hispanoamericanos* 250–52 (1970–71): 664–77.

——. *M. Seoane La introducción en España del sistema sanitario liberal (1791–1870).* Madrid: Ministerio de Sanidad y Consumo, 1984.

——, Luís García Ballester and Pilar Faus Sevilla. *Medicina y sociedad en la España del siglo XIX.* Madrid: Sociedad de Estudios y Publicaciones, 1964.

McGrew, Roderick E. *Russia and the Cholera 1823–1832.* Madison: University of Wisconsin Press, 1965.

Madariaga de la Campa, Benito. *Pérez Galdós: Biografía Santanderina.* pról. Joaquín Casalduero, cronología por Celia Valbuena de Madariaga. Santander: Institución Cultural de Cantabria, 1979.

Magnan, Valentin. *De l'alcoolisme des diverse formes du délire alcoolique et de leur traitment.* Paris: Adrien Delahaye, 1874.

——. and Paul Legrain. *Les dégénérés.* Paris: Rueff et Cie., 1895.

"Los manicomios de España." *El siglo médico* 30 Dec. 1888: 846–47.

Marañón, Gregorio. "La ciencia española y su contribución al mundo actual." *Obras Completas.* Vol. 2. *Discursos.* Madrid: Espasa-Calpe 1966. 483–90.

——. "Contestación al discurso de recepción, en la Real Academia Española, de Don Pío Baroja." *Obras Completas.* Vol. 2. *Discursos.* Madrid: Espasa-Calpe 1966. 319–29.

——. *Elogio y nostalgia de Toledo.* 2nd ed. Madrid: Espasa-Calpe S.A., 1951.

——. "La pasión sobre Ferrán." *Obras Completas.* Vol. 4. *Artículos y otros trabajos.* Madrid: Espasa-Calpe, S.A., 1968. 859–61.

——. "Galdós íntimo." *Obras completas.* Vol. 4. *Artículos y otros trabajos.* Madrid: Espasa-Calpe, S.A., 1968. 27–29.

——. "Psiquiatras de España." *Obras Completas.* Vol. 9. *Ensayos.* Madrid: Espasa-Calpe, S.A., 1973. 82–87.

——. "Menéndez Pelayo y España." *Obras Completas.* Vol. 9. *Tiempo viejo y tiempo nuevo.* Madrid: Espasa-Calpe, S.A., 1973. 430–44.

——. "Vocación y Ética." *Obras completas.* Vol. 9. *Vocación y ética y otros Ensayos.* Madrid: Espasa-Calpe, S.A., 1973. 327–45.

Marco, Luís. *La difteria en España y en Madrid.* Madrid: Est. Tip, Enrique Teodoro, 1888.

Martínez y Suárez, Fermín. *Lactancia bajo todas sus manifestaciones*. Madrid: R. Velasco, 1887.

Mateos Fernández, Juan Carlos. "Cuestión de honor. Los periodistas se baten en duelo." *Historia y comunicación social* 3 (1998): 232–41.

Maudsley, Henry. "Materialism and its Lessons." *The Fortnightly Review*" 26 (1879): 244–60.

——. "Los medios de preservarse de la locura (part 1)." *Revista Europea* 24 Jan. 1875: 407–15.

——. *The Physiology and Pathology of Mind* (1867). London: Routledge, 1993.

——. "Sex in Mind and Education." *Popular Science Monthly* June 1874: 198–215.

"M.D." "Confederación médica española." *Boletín de medicina, cirugía y farmacia* 4 (1849): 25–26.

Méndez, Gabino and Juan Pereda. *Manual del destilador, licorista y perfumista: comprende un tratado teórico-práctico de destilación; la manera de fabricar toda clase de aguardiente, aguas destiladas, aceites esenciales*. Paris: Lib. Rosa y Bouret, 1858.

Méndez Álvaro, Francisco. *De la actividad humana en sus relaciones con la salud y el gobierno de los pueblos: Discurso leido ante la Real Academia de Medicina de Madrid [...] el año de 1864*. Madrid: M. Rojas, 1864.

——. "Fragmentos de un curioso informe relativo al estado de las profesiones médicas en España ..." *El siglo médico* 23 Nov. 1862: 738–40; 30 Nov. 1862: 754–59.

Menéndez Pelayo, Marcelino. "Benito Pérez Galdós considerado como novelista." *Estudios de crítica literaria*. Madrid: Tip. Revista de Archivos, 1908. 83–128.

Mesa, Rafael de. *Don Benito Pérez Galdós: Su familia.-sus mocedades, su senectud*. Madrid: Juan Pueyo Luna, 1920.

Mesonero Romanos, Ramón de. "Antes, ahora, y después." (1837) *Escenas y tipos matritenses*. Ed. Enrique Rubio Cremades. Madrid: Cátedra, 1993. 332–51.

Meyer, Édouard. *Traité pratique des maladies des yeux*. 2nd ed. Paris: G. Masson, 1880.

Monlau, Pedro Felipe. *Elementos de higiene privada o Arte de conservar la salud del individuo*. 4th ed. Madrid: Lib. Moya y Plaza, 1870.

——. *Higiene del matrimonio*. 5th ed., Madrid: Imp. Esteoriotip. Galvano. Aribau y Cª., 1881.

——. *Remedios del pauperismo. Memoria para optar al premio ofrecido por la Sociedad Económica Matritenses el 1 de mayo de 1845*. Madrid: Sociedad Económica, 1846.

Monmeneu, José. *La enfermedades infecciosas en Madrid*. Madrid: Admin. Revista Med. y Cir. Pract., 1894.

Montesinos, José F. *Galdós*. 3 vols. Madrid: Editorial Castalia, 1968.

Moreau (de Tours), Jacques-Joseph. *La psychologie morbide dans ses rapports avec la philosophie de l'histoire ou de l'influence des névropathies sur le dynamisme intellectuel*. Paris: Lib. Victor Masson, 1859.

Morel, B.A. *Traité de dégénérescences physiques, intellectuelles et morales de l'espèce humaine et des causes qui produisent ces variétés maldives*. Paris: Ballière, 1857.

——. *Traité de maladies mentales*. Paris: Victor Masson, 1860.

Moreno Fernández, Jose. "La tisis tuberculosa bajo el concepto social." *Conferencias científicas leídas por los profesores en la Escuela de Medicina de Sevilla. Curso 1888–1889*. Sevilla: Imp. Díaz y Carbello, 1889. 5–11, 13–20; *Estudios medicosociales sobre la tuberculosis en la España de la Restauración*. Ed. Jorge Molero Mesa. Madrid: Ministerio de Sanidad y Consumo, 1987. 53–67.

Morens, David M., Jeffery K. Taubenberger, and Anthony S. Fauci. "Predominant Role of Bacterial Pneumonia as a Cause of Death in Pandemic Influenza: Implications for Pandemic Influenza Preparedness." *The Journal of Infectious Diseases* 198 (2008): 1–9.

Morote, Luis. "En Santander oyendo á Pérez Galdós." *Heraldo de Madrid* 31 Aug. 1903: 1.

Morris, R.J. *Cholera 1832. The Social Response to an Epidemic*. London: Croom Helm, 1976.

"Muerte de un gran español." *El Figaro* 4 Jan. 1920: 5–6.

Munoa Roiz, J.L. "Historia de la oftalmología española contemporánea." *Cuadernos de Historia de la Medicina Española* 111.1 (1964): 41–87.

——, and J.L. Cotallo. "Enseñanza y ejercicio de la oftalmología" J.L. Cotallo de Cáceres, E. Hernández Benito, J.L. Munoa Roiz and G. Leoz de la Fuente. *Historia de la oftalmología española*. Madrid: Sociedad Española de Oftalmología, 1993. 181–203.

Nieto Serrano, Matías. "Discurso leído por el secretario perpetuo Dr. D. Matías Nieto Serrano en la sesión inaugural de este año." *El siglo médico* 23 Apr. 1893: 270–71; 30 Apr. 1893: 286–87.

Nimitz, Michael. *Humor in Galdós: A Study of the "Novelas contemporáneas."* New Haven: Yale University Press, 1968.

Nuttall, G.H.F. and G.S. Graham-Smith. Ed. *The Bacteriology of Diphtheria*. Cambridge: Cambridge University Press, 1908.

O'Dwyer, Joseph. "Intubation in Croup and other Acute and Chronic Forms of Stenosis of the Larynx." C.E. Billington and Joseph O'Dwyer. *Diphtheria its Nature and Treatment and Intubation in Croup*. New York: William Wood, 1889. 265–308.

Ondráček, O., and M. Lokaj. "Visual outcome after congenital cataract surgery: Long-term clinical results." *Scripta Medica (Brno)*. 76.2 (2003): 95–102.

Ortega, Manuel L. *El doctor Pulido*. Madrid: Editorial Ibero-Africano-Americano, 1922.

Ortega Munilla, José. "La vuelta del año." *La ilustración artística* 3 Nov. 1884: 2.

Ortiz-Armengol, Pedro. *Vida de Galdós*. Barcelona: Crítica, 1996.

Parrot, Joseph M.J. "Nourricerie de l'hospice des enfants assistées." *Bulletin de l'Académie de Médecine* 11 (1882): 839–53.

——. "Le Rachitis et la Syphilis héréditaire." *Transactions of the Seventh Session of the International Medical Congress London 2nd-9th August 1881*. Ed. Sir William MacCormac and George H. Makins. Vol. 4. London: J.W. Kolckmann, 1881. 35–40, 57.

Pattison, Walter T. *El naturalismo español. Historia externa de un movimiento literario* Madrid: Editorial Gredos, 1965.

Payan, Mr. *Del empleo del yoduro de potasio en las enfermedades sifilíticas*. Trans. José Dias Oyuelos. Burgos: Imp. Lit. lib. de Azpiazu, 1847.

Pearce, J.M.S. "A brief history of the clinical thermometer." *Quarterly Journal of Medicine* 95.4 (2002): 251–52.

Pérez Bautista, Florencio L. *El tema de la enfermedad en la novela realista española*. Salamanca, Universidad de Salamanca, 1972.

Pérez Galdós, Benito. *El amigo Manso*. Ed. Francisco Caudet. Madrid: Cátedra, 2001.

——. *Ángel Guerra*. Madrid: Lib. Casa Ed. Hernando, S.A., 1970.

——. *Los artículos de Galdós en "La Nación," 1865–1866*. Ed. y estudio prelim. William H. Shoemaker. Madrid: Insula, 1972.

——. *La de Bringas*. 5th ed. Ed. Alda Blanco and Carlos Blanco Aguinaga. Madrid: Cátedra, 1997.

——. "Carta a Leopoldo Alas." 6 Apr. 1885. *Galdós: Lectura de una vida*. Ed. Alfonso Armas Ayala. Santa Cruz de Tenerife: Servicio de Publicaciones de la Caja General de Ahorros de Canarias, 1989. 229–30.

——. "Carta a La Prensa." 18 Dec. 1893. William H. Shoemaker. *Las cartas desconocidas de Galdós en "La Prensa" de Buenos Aires*. Madrid: Ediciones Cultura Hispánica, 1973. 505.

——. *Las cartas desconocidas de Galdós en "La Prensa" de Buenos Aires*. Ed. and preliminary study William H. Shoemaker. Madrid: Ediciones Cultura Hispánica, 1973.

——. "El crimen del cura Galeote III, 9 Oct. 1886." in Benito Pérez Galdós. *Obras Inéditas vol. VII Cronicón (1886–1890)*. Ed. and prol. Alberto Ghiraldo. Madrid: Renacimiento, (n.d.) 176–82.

——. *La desheredada*. 2nd ed. Ed. Germán Guillón. Madrid: Cátedra, 2003.

——. *El doctor Centeno*. Ed. Isabel Ramón Ramón. Cáceres: Universidad de Extremadura, 2008.

——. *Un faccioso más y algunos frailes menos*. Madrid: Librería y Casa Editorial Hernando S.A., 1948.

——. *La familia de León Roch*. Ed. Íñigo Sánchez Llama. Madrid: Cátedra, 2003.

——. *Fortuna y Jacinta*. vol. 1. 7th ed. Ed. Francisco Caudet. Madrid: Cátedra, 2002; vol. 2. 5th ed. Ed. Francisco Caudet. Madrid: Cátedra, 1999.

——. *Lo prohibido*. Ed. James Whiston. Madrid: Cátedra, 2001.
——. *Marianela*. Ed. Francisco Caudet. Madrid: Cátedra, 2003.
——. *Marianela*. Ed. Joaquín Casalduero. Madrid: Cátedra, 1983.
——. *Memorias de un desmemoriado*. (1915) *Crónica de Madrid*. Ed. and prol. Juan Van-Halen. Madrid: Comunidad de Madrid. Consejería de Educación, 2004.
——. *Miau*. 6th ed. Ed. Franciso Javier Díez de Revenga. Madrid: Cátedra, 2007.
——. *Las novelas de Torquemada: Torquemada en la hoguera*. Madrid: Alianza Editorial 1970.
——. *Obras Inéditas: Crónicon (1883–1886)*. Vol. 6. Ord. and prol. Alberto Ghiraldo. Madrid: Renacimiento, 1924.
——. *Obras Inéditas: Crónicon (1886–1890)*. Vol. 7. Ord. and prol. Alberto Ghiraldo. Madrid: Renacimiento, undated.
——. "Observaciones sobre la novela contemporánea en España." *Revista de España* 15.57 (1870): 162–172.
——. "Prólogo." Manuel Tolosa Latour. *Niñerías*. Madrid: Tipografía Manuel Ginés Hernández, 1889. i–xii.
Pick, Daniel. *Faces of Degeneration: A European Disorder, c. 1848-c. 1918*. Cambridge: Cambridge University Press, 1989.
Pinel, Philippe. *Traité médico-philosophique sur l'aliénation mentale*. 2nd ed. Paris: J. Ant. Brosson, 1809.
"¡Pobres médicos rurales!" *El genio médico-quirúrico* 15 Aug. 1885: 456.
Poncet de Cluny, F. "Tetanus." *Nouveau dictionnaire de médecine et de chirurgie pratiques* Vol. 35. Paris: Baillière et fils, 1885. 360–465.
Prichard, James C. *A Treatise on Insanity and Other Disorders Affecting the Mind*. Philadelphia: Carey and Hart, 1837.
Pulido Fernández, Ángel. "Barcelona médica II." *El siglo médico* 16 Dec. 1888: 802–03.
——. *Bosquejos médico-sociales para la mujer*. Madrid: Víctor Saiz, 1876.
——. "Conflictos entre la frenopatía y el código. Carta dirigida al Dr. Esquerdo." J. Guislain. *Lecciones orales sobre las frenopatías ó tratado teórico práctico de las enfermedades mentales*. 2 vols. 2nd ed. Trans. M. Carreras Sanchis and J. Torres Fabregat. Madrid: Imp. Enrique Teodoro, 1881. v–xl.
——. "Dirección General de Sanidad. Circular." *El siglo médico* 15 Jun. 1902: 879–90.
——. *Locos delincuentes [...] Estado actual de la ciencia frenopática y sus relaciones con el derecho penal*. Madrid: Imp. de la Revista de Legislación, 1883; Luís Maristany, "Lombroso y España: Nuevas consideraciones." *Anales de Literatura Española* 2 (1983): 361–81. 371.
——. "Locos que no lo parecen." *El siglo médico* 10 Feb. 1881: 84–86.
——. "Los manicomios de España: El de Santa Isabel de Leganés." *El siglo médico* 17 Feb. 1889: 101–02.

——. "Nuevo manicomio." *El anfiteatro anatómico español* 31 May 1877: 141–42.
——. *Sanidad pública en España y ministerio social de las clases médicas*. Madrid: Imp. Enrique Teodoro y Alonso, 1902.
——. "Tras de la inoculación colerígena (impresiones de un viaje á Valencia)." *El siglo médico* 3 May 1885: 273–78.
—— and Manuel Tolosa Latour. "De Carabanchel al paraíso (recuerdos de un manicomio)." *El siglo médico* 29 (1882): 336–37, 433–34, 448–49, 466–67, 497–99, 514–15, 529–30.
Pulido Martín, Ángel. *El dr. Pulido y su época*. pról. Jacinto Benavente. Madrid: F. Domenich, S.A., 1945.
"Query: Do vegetables produce cholera?" *London Medical Gazette* 24 Nov. 1833: 261–64.
Quétel, Claude. *The History of Syphilis*. Trans. Judith Braddock and Brian Pike. Baltimore: Johns Hopkins University Press, 1990.
Ray Lankester, E. "The Truth about Koch's Cholera Germ." *Pall Mall Gazette* 6 Oct. 1884: 1–2.
Régis, Emmanuel. *La folie à deux ou folie simultanée avec observations recueillies à la Clinique de Pathologie Mentale (Asile Sainte-Anne)*. Paris: J-B Ballière et Fils, 1880.
Reglamento de la Inspección de Salubridad Pública en sus secciones de higiene de las nodrizas y de la prostitución. Madrid: Imp. del Hospicio, 1877.
Renaudin, M. le D^r^. "De l'alcoolisme chronique par M. le Dr Magnus Huss." *Annales Médico-Psychologiques* 5 (1853): 60–88.
Ribbans, Geoffrey. *History and Fiction in Galdós's Narratives*. Oxford: Clarendon Press, 1993.
——. *Pérez Galdós: Fortunata y Jacinta*. London: Grant and Cutler Ltd., 1977.
Ricard, Robert. "Tolosa Latour, el P. Lerchundi y *La loca de la casa*." *Anales galdosianos* 3 (1968): 87–90.
Rivers, W.C. "The Atavistic-Degenerative Diathesis of Tuberculosis." *The Lancet* 20 Jan. 1923: 120–24.
Rolleston, J.D. "Bretonneau: His Life and Work." *Journal of the Royal Society of Medicine* 18 (1925): 1–12.
Rosenau, Milton. *The Milk Question*. Boston: Houghton Mifflin Company, 1912.
Rosenberg, Charles E. "Florence Nightingale on contagion: The hospital as moral universe." *Explaining epidemics and other studies in the history of medicine*. Cambridge: Cambridge University Press, 1992. 90–108.
——. "The Place of George M. Beard in Nineteenth-Century Psychiatry." *Bulletin of the History of Medicine* 36 (1962): 245–59.
Roura, José. *Memoria sobre los vinos y su destilación y sobre los aceites*. Barcelona: Imp. J. Olivares y Gavarró, 1839.

Routh, C.H.F. *Infant Feeding and its Influence on Life*. 3rd ed. London: J. and A. Churchill, 1876.
Rubin, Walter. "Galdós y la medicina." *Atlántida* 8.43 (1970): 68–80.
Ruiz, Mario E. "El idealismo platónico en 'Marianela' de Galdós." *Hispania* 53.4 (1970): 870–80.
Sacks, Oliver. "Face-blind." *The New Yorker* 30 Aug. 2010: 36–43.
Salillas, Rafael. "Los locos delincuentes en España." *Revista General de Legislación y Jurisprudencia* 94 (1899): 117–42.
San Martín, Alejandro. *Influjo del descubrimiento del Nuevo Mundo en las ciencias Médicas*. Madrid: Est. Tip. Sucesores de Rivadeneyra, 1892.
Sánchez Vázquez, V., and T. Guijarro Granados. "Apuntes para una historia de las instituciones de menores en España." *Revista de la Asociación Española de Neuropsiquiatría* 22.84 (2002): 121–38.
Sanson y Portillo, José. "La profesión médica en España." *El siglo médico* 52 installments from 9 Sep. 1877 to 24 Nov. 1878.
Santero, Franciso Javier. *Elementos de higiene privada y pública*. Madrid: El Cosmos Editorial, 1885.
Sarasúa, Carmen. *Criados, nodrizas y amos: El servicio doméstico en la formación del mercado de trabajo madrileño, 1758–1868*. Madrid: Siglo Veintiuno de España Editores S.A., 1994.
Savoyen, L. *Nouvelles études philosophiques sur la dégénération physique et morale de l'homme*. Paris: J. Hamel, 1854.
Scanlon, Geraldine M. "Problema social y krausismo en '*Marianela*.'" *Actas del Tercer Congreso Internacional de Estudios Galdosianos I*. Las Palmas: Cabildo Insular, (1989): 81–95.
Schmidt, Ruth. *Cartas entre dos amigos del teatro*. Madrid: Cabildo Insular de Gran Canaria, 1969.
Schnepf, Michael A. "The Naturalistic Content of the *La desheredada* Manuscript." *Anales galdosianos* 24 (1989): 53–59.
Scott, D.F. "The Discovery of anti-epileptic drugs." *Journal of the History of the Neurosciences* 1 (1992): 111–18.
Seguin, Eduardo C. "Notes on Spanish Asylums for the Insane." *Journal of Nervous and Mental Disease* 3 (1883): 379–420. [Appeared in translation 1884: "Apuntes sobre los manicomios españoles." *Primer certamen frenopático español: celebrado en los días 25, 26, 27 y 28 de septiembre de 1883 en el manicomio Nueva-Belén*. Ed. José Giné y Partagas. Barcelona: Est. Tip. La Academia, 1884.]
Serrano Fatigati, Enrique. *Alimentos adulterados y defunciones*. Madrid: Imp. El Día Lucas Polo, 1883.
Shoemaker, William H. "Cómo era Galdós?" *Anales galdosianos* 8 (1973): 5–21.

——. "Estudio preliminar." Benito Pérez Galdós. *Las cartas desconocidas de Galdós en "La Prensa" de Buenos Aires*. Madrid: Ediciones Cultura Hispánica, 1973. 7–40.

Sieveking, Edward H. "Analysis of fifty-two cases of epilepsy observed by the author." *The Lancet* 69.1760 (1857): 527–28.

Smith, Michael Anthony. "Medicine in the Works of Benito Pérez Galdós." Diss. (M.A.) University of Birmingham, 1977.

Snow, John. *On the Mode of Communication of Cholera*. 2nd ed. London: John Churchill, 1855.

Stannard, Michael W. "Maximiliano Rubín and the Context of Galdós's Medical Knowledge." *Anales galdosianos* 48 (2013): 97–111.

——. *The Theme of Degeneration in the Work of Benito Pérez Galdós: A Study of Four Naturalist Novels*. Saarbrücken: Lambert Academic Publishing, 2012.

Sutherland, John. *Report of the General Board of Health on the Epidemic of Cholera of 1848 and 1849*. London: HMSO, 1850.

Sutton, Thomas. *Tracts on Delirium Tremens, on Peritonitis and on Some Other Inflammatory Affections, and on the Gout*. London: Thomas Underwood, 1813.

Tejada y España, Félix. "¿Es arte, oficio ó sacerdocio la profesión médica?" *El genio médico-quirúrgico* 15 Jan. 1881: 14.

——. "La conferencia del Dr. Esquerdo sobre Garayo (Saca-Mantecas)." [Revista de la Semana] *El genio médico-quirúrgico* 31 Jan. 1881: 45–46.

——. "Gran Conferencia: Locos que no lo parecen." *El genio médico-quirúrgico* 15 Mar. 1880: 144–45.

——. "La profesión." [Sección profesional] *El genio médico-quirúrgico* 7 Jan. 1881: 4–5.

Thompson, William (Lord Kelvin). "On the age of the Sun's Heat." *Macmillan's Magazine* 5 Mar. 1862: 288–93.

Tolosa Latour, Manuel. *Discurso pronunciado en el Congreso Internacional para la Protección de la Infancia*. Madrid: Enrique Teodoro, 1883.

——. *Instrucciones populares para evitar la propagación y estragos de la difteria, garrotillo, anginas gangrenosas, crup*. Madrid: Oficinas de la Sociedad Española de Higiene, 1886.

——. *El Niño*. Madrid: La Gaceta Universal, 1880.

——. *La protección médica al niño desválido*. Madrid: Imp. Sres. García y Caravera, 1881.

——. "Siluetas contemporáneas: Esquerdo." *El Imparcial* 27 Sep. 1880: 2.

——. (El doctor Fausto) "Siluetas contemporáneas: Pérez Galdós." *La Época* 26 Mar. 1883: 3.

Trotter, Thomas. *An Essay, Medical, Philosophical, and Chemical, on Drunkenness and its Effects on the Human Body*. London: T.N. Longman and O. Rees, 1804.

Tuñon de Lara, Manuel. *Medio siglo de cultura española*. 3rd ed. Madrid: Editorial Tecnos, 1973.

Udwadia, Farokh E. *Tetanus*. Bombay: Oxford University Press, 1994.
Ullman, Joan C. and George H. Allison "Galdós as Psychiatrist in Fortunata y Jacinta." *Anales galdosianos* 9 (1974): 7–36.
Unamuno, Miguel de. "La sociedad galdosiana." *Obras completes, Vol. 3 Nuevos ensayos*. Madrid: Escelicer, 1968. 1203–04.
Van Deusen, E.H. *Observations on a Form of Nervous Prostration (Neurasthenia) Culminating in Insanity*. Lansing: W.S. George and Co., 1869.
Vaphiades, Michael S., Gastone G. Celesia, and Mitchell G. Brigell. "Positive spontaneous visual phenomena limited to the hemianopic field in lesions of central visual pathways." *Neurology* 47 (1996): 408–17.
Varela de Montes, José. *Preceptos y consejos sobre el cólera*. Santiago: Est. Tip. Manuel Mirás, 1865.
Vera, Jaime. *Estudio clínico de la parálisis general de los enajenados*. pról. José María Esquerdo. Madrid: Moya y Plaza, 1880.
Vezalde, Ramón. "¡Meditamos!" *El siglo médico* 3 Feb. 1878. 69. Agustín Albarracín Teulón. "La asociaciones médicas en España durante el siglo XIX." *Cuadernos de historia de la medicina española* 10 (1971): 157.
——. "La profesión." *El siglo médico* 18 Oct. 1874: 657–59.
Vidal Parellada, Assumpciò. *Luís Simarro y su tiempo*. Madrid: Consejo Superior de Investigaciones Científicas, 2007.
Villasante, Olga. "Las instituciones psiquiátricas madrileñas en el período de entresiglos: Asistencia pública frente a sanatorios privados." *Frenia* 5.1 (2005): 69–99.
——. "La introducción del concepto de 'Parálisis General Progresiva' en la psiquiatría decimonónica española." *Asclepio* 52.1 (2000): 53–72.
——. and Rafael Huertas. "El manicomio del Dr. Esquerdo: entre la promoción empresarial y la legitimación científica." *SISO/SAUDE. Boletín da Asociación Galega de Saúde Mental.* 32 (1999): 27–34.
Viñeta-Bellaserra, José. *Profilaxia de la sífilis en el niño y en la nodriza por medio de la lactancia animal, particularmente en las maternidades y casas de expósitos*. Barcelona: Tip. Casa Provincial de Caridad, 1889.
——. *La sífilis como hecho social punible y como una de las causas de la degeneración de la raza humana discurso pronunciado en la Sociedad Económica Graciense de Amigos del País en la sesión del 8 de marzo de 1885 por J. Viñeta-Bellaserra*. Barcelona: Est. Tip. Edit. La Academia, 1886.
Voelcker, Augustus. "On Milk." *Journal of the Royal Agricultural Society of England* 24 (1863): 286–320.
Vozmediano Hidalgo, María Luisa. "Las ciencias médicas a través de las novelas de D. Benito Pérez Galdós." Diss. Universidad Complutense, Facultad de Farmacia, 1981.

Wallace, William. "Treatment of the venereal disease by the hydriodate of potash, or iodide of potassium." *The Lancet* 36.2 (1835): 5–11.

Walton, Leslie B. *Pérez Galdós and the Spanish Novel of the Nineteenth Century*. London: J.M. Dent and Sons Ltd., 1927.

——. "La psicología anormal en la obra de Galdós." *Boletin del Instituto Español* 4 (1948): 10–13.

Warlomont, E. "Nystagmus." *Dictionnaire Encyclopédique des Sciences Médicales*. Vol. 13. Paris: G. Masson, 1879: 825–53.

Wecker, L. de. *Cirujía ocular*. Madrid: Imp. de Enrique Teodoro, 1879.

Welch, Francis J. "Aortic Aneurysm in the Army, and the conditions associated with it." *The Lancet* 27 Nov. 1875: 769–71.

Whiston, James. "Introducción." Benito Pérez Galdós *Lo prohibido*. Madrid: Cátedra, (2001): 11–126.

Wiesel, Torsten N. "Postnatal development of the visual cortex and the influence of environment." *Nature* 299.14 (1982): 583–91.

Wigan, A.L. *The Duality of Mind*. London: Longman, Brown, Green, and Longmans, 1844.

Willey, Jack R. "The Médico as a Literary Personage in the Works of Benito Pérez Galdós." Diss. University of Illinois, 1969.

Yvaren, Próspero. *De las metamórfosis de la sífilis. Investigaciones acerca del diagnóstico de las enfermedades que la sífilis puede simular y acerca de la sífilis latente*. Trans. José Ametller y Viñas. Madrid: Imp. Manuel Alvarez, 1860.

Index

Hispanic Studies: Culture and Ideas

Edited by
Claudio Canaparo

This series aims to publish studies in the arts, humanities and social sciences, the main focus of which is the Hispanic World. The series invites proposals with interdisciplinary approaches to Hispanic culture in fields such as the history of concepts and ideas, the sociology of culture, the evolution of visual arts, the critique of literature, and the uses of historiography. It is not confined to a particular historical period.

Monographs as well as collected papers are welcome in English or Spanish.

Those interested in contributing to the series are invited to write with either the synopsis of a subject already in typescript or with a detailed project outline to either Professor Claudio Canaparo, Department of Iberian and Latin American Studies, School of Arts, Birkbeck College, 43 Gordon Square, London WC1H 0PD, UK, c.canaparo@sllc.bbk.ac.uk, or Peter Lang Ltd, oxford@peterlang.com.

Vol. 1 Antonio Sánchez
Postmodern Spain. A Cultural Analysis of 1980s–1990s Spanish Culture. 220 pages. 2007.
ISBN 978-3-03910-914-2

Vol. 2 Geneviève Fabry y Claudio Canaparo (eds.)
El enigma de lo real. Las fronteras del realismo en la narrativa del siglo XX. 275 pages. 2007.
ISBN 978-3-03910-893-0

Vol. 3 William Rowlandson
Reading Lezama's *Paradiso*. 290 pages. 2007.
ISBN 978-3-03910-751-3

Vol. 4 Fernanda Peñaloza, Jason Wilson and Claudio Canaparo (eds)
Patagonia. Myths and Realities. 277 pages. 2010.
ISBN 978-3-03910-917-3

Vol. 5 Xon de Ros
Primitivismo y Modernismo. El legado de María Blanchard.
238 pages. 2007.
ISBN 978-3-03910-937-1

Vol. 6 Sergio Plata
Visions of Applied Mathematics. Strategy and Knowledge.
284 pages. 2007.
ISBN 978-3-03910-923-4

Vol. 7 Annick Louis
Borges ante el fascismo. 374 pages. 2007.
ISBN 978-3-03911-005-6

Vol. 8 Helen Oakley
From Revolution to Migration. A Study of Contemporary Cuban and Cuban-American Crime Fiction. 200 pages. 2012.
ISBN 978-3-03911-021-6

Vol. 9 Thea Pitman
Mexican Travel Writing. 209 pages. 2008.
ISBN 978-3-03911-020-9

Vol. 10 Francisco J. Borge
A New World for a New Nation. The Promotion of America in Early Modern England. 240 pages. 2007.
ISBN 978-3-03911-070-4

Vol. 11 Helena Buffery, Stuart Davis and Kirsty Hooper (eds)
Reading Iberia. Theory/History/Identity. 229 pages. 2007.
ISBN 978-3-03911-109-1

Vol. 12 Matías Bruera
Mapping the Tasteland. Explorations in Food and Wine in Argentinean and European Culture. 240 pages. 2014.
ISBN 978-3-03911-345-3

Vol. 13 Angela Romero-Astvaldsson
La obra narrativa de David Viñas. La nueva inflexión de *Prontuario* y *Claudia Conversa*. 300 pages. 2007.
ISBN 978-3-03911-100-8

Vol. 14 Aaron Kahn
The Ambivalence of Imperial Discourse. Cervantes's *La Numancia* within the 'Lost Generation' of Spanish Drama (1570–90).
243 pages. 2008.
ISBN 978-3-03911-098-8

Vol. 15 Turid Hagene
Negotiating Love in Post-Revolutionary Nicaragua. The role of love in the reproduction of gender asymmetry. 341 pages. 2008.
ISBN 978-3-03911-011-7

Vol. 16 Yolanda Rodríguez Pérez
The Dutch Revolt through Spanish Eyes. Self and Other in historical and literary texts of Golden Age Spain (c. 1548–1673). 346 pages. 2008.
ISBN 978-3-03911-136-7

Vol. 17 Stanley Black (ed.)
Juan Goytisolo. Territories of Life and Writing. 202 pages. 2007.
ISBN 978-3-03911-324-8

Vol. 18 María T. Sánchez
The Problems of Literary Translation. A Study of the Theory and Practice of Translation from English into Spanish. 269 pages. 2009.
ISBN 978-3-03911-326-2

Vol. 19 Aino Linda Rinhaug
Fernando Pessoa. A Ludicrous Self. *Forthcoming*.
ISBN 978-3-03911-909-7

Vol. 20 Ana Cruz García
Re(de-)generando identidades. Locura, feminidad y liberalización en Elena Garro, Susana Pagano, Ana Castillo y María Amparo Escandón.
259 pages. 2009.
ISBN 978-3-03911-524-2

Vol. 21 Idoya Puig (ed.)
Tradition and Modernity. Cervantes's Presence in Spanish Contemporary Literature. 221 pages. 2009.
ISBN 978-3-03911-526-6

Vol. 22 Charlotte Lange
Modos de parodia. Guillermo Cabrera Infante, Reinaldo Arenas, Jorge Ibargüengoitia y José Agustín. 252 pages. 2008.
ISBN 978-3-03911-554-9

Vol. 23 Claudio Canaparo
Geo-epistemology. Latin America and the Location of Knowledge. 284 pages. 2009.
ISBN 978-3-03911-573-0

Vol. 24 Jesús López-Peláez Casellas
"Honourable Murderers". El concepto del honor en *Othello* de Shakespeare y en los "dramas de honor" de Calderón. 321 pages. 2009.
ISBN 978-3-03911-825-0

Vol. 25 Marian Womack and Jennifer Wood (eds)
Beyond the Back Room. New Perspectives on Carmen Martín Gaite. 336 pages. 2011.
ISBN 978-3-03911-827-4

Vol. 26 Manuela Palacios and Laura Lojo (eds)
Writing Bonds. Irish and Galician Contemporary Women Poets. 232 pages. 2009.
ISBN 978-3-03911-834-2

Vol. 27 Myriam Osorio
Agencia femenina, agencia narrativa. Una lectura feminista de la obra en prosa de Albalucía Ángel. 180 pages. 2010.
ISBN 978-3-03911-893-3

Vol. 28 *Forthcoming*

Vol. 29 Soledad Pérez-Abadín Barro
Cortázar y Che Guevara. Lectura de *Reunión*. 182 pages. 2010.
ISBN 978-3-03911-919-6

Vol. 30 Gonzalo Pasamar
Apologia and Criticism. Historians and the History of Spain, 1500–2000. 301 pages. 2010.
ISBN 978-3-03911-920-2

Vol. 31 Victoria Carpenter (ed.)
(Re)Collecting the Past. History and Collective Memory in Latin American Narrative. 315 pages. 2010.
ISBN 978-3-03911-928-8

Vol. 32 Geneviève Fabry, Ilse Logie y Pablo Decock (eds.)
Los imaginarios apocalípticos en la literatura hispanoamericana contemporánea. 472 pages. 2010.
ISBN 978-3-03911-937-0

Vol. 33 Julian Vigo
Performative Bodies, Hybrid Tongues. Race, Gender, Sex and Modernity in Latin America and the Maghreb. 391 pages. 2010.
ISBN 978-3-03911-951-6

Vol. 34 Heike Pintor Pirzkall
La cooperación alemana al desarrollo. Factores condicionantes de su transformación en la década de los noventa y su impacto en América Latina. 374 pages. 2010.
ISBN 978-3-0343-0107-7

Vol. 35 Arturo Casas and Ben Bollig (eds)
Resistance and Emancipation. Cultural and Poetic Practices. 419 pages. 2011.
ISBN 978-3-0343-0160-2

Vol. 36 Pablo Decock
Las figuras paradójicas de César Aira. Un estudio semiótico y axiológico de la estereotipia y la autofiguración. 344 pages. 2014.
ISBN 978-3-0343-0169-5

Vol. 37 Guillermo Olivera
Laboratorios de la mediatización. La experimentación con materiales mediáticos, la teoría y la crítica cultural argentina, 1965–1978.
364 pages. 2011.
ISBN 978-3-0343-0201-2

Vol. 38 Guy Baron
Gender in Cuban Cinema. From the Modern to the Postmodern.
334 pages. 2011.
ISBN 978-3-0343-0229-6

Vol. 39 Claudio Canaparo
El imaginario Patagonia. Ensayo acerca de la evolución conceptual del espacio. 576 pages. 2011.
ISBN 978-3-0343-0287-6

Vol. 40 Inmaculada Murcia Serrano
Agua y destino. Introducción a la estética de Ramón Gaya.
220 pages. 2011.
ISBN 978-3-0343-0251-7

Vol. 41 Bill Richardson
Borges and Space. 266 pages. 2012.
ISBN 978-3-0343-0246-3

Vol. 42 *Forthcoming*

Vol. 43 Ann Frost
The Galician Works of Ramón del Valle-Inclán. Patterns of Repetition and Continuity. 241 pages. 2010.
ISBN 978-3-0343-0242-5

Vol. 44 Milagros López-Peláez Casellas
What About the Girls? Estrategias narrativas de resistencia en la primera literatura chicana. 265 pages. 2012.
ISBN 978-3-0343-0264-7

Vol. 45 Bill Richardson and Lorraine Kelly (eds)
Power, Place and Representation. Contested Sites of Dependence and Independence in Latin America. 268 pages. 2012.
ISBN 978-3-0343-0710-9

Vol. 46 Patricia D'Allemand
José María Samper. Nación y cultura en el siglo XIX colombiano.
177 pages. 2012.
ISBN 978-3-0343-0288-3

Vol. 47 *Forthcoming*

Vol. 48 Emilio Rosales
Baroja. La novela como laberinto. 163 pages. 2012.
ISBN 978-3-0343-0774-1

Vol. 49 Kristine Vanden Berghe
Las novelas de la rebelión zapatista. 171 pages. 2012.
ISBN 978-3-0343-0779-6

Vol. 50 William Rowlandson
Borges, Swedenborg and Mysticism. 267 pages. 2013.
ISBN 978-3-0343-0811-3

Vol. 51 Elena Rodríguez-Guridi
Exégesis del "error". Una reinterpretación de la praxis de escritura en *Libro de la vida*, *Novelas ejemplares* y *Desengaños amorosos*.
175 pages. 2013.
ISBN 978-3-0343-0817-5

Vol. 52 Eva Bru-Domínguez
Beyond Containment. Corporeality in Mercè Rodoreda's Literature.
235 pages. 2013
ISBN 978-3-0343-0888-5

Vol. 53 Gabriele Andreozzi (ed.)
Desaparición. Argentina's Human Rights Trials. 355 pages. 2014.
ISBN 978-3-0343-0857-1

Vol. 54 Mel Boland
Displacement in Isabel Allende's Fiction, 1982–2000.
212 pages. 2013.
ISBN 978-3-0343-0932-5

Vol. 55 Eduardo Tasis Moratinos
El exilio en la poesía de Tomás Segovia y Angelina Muñiz Huberman.
234 pages. 2014.
ISBN 978-3-0343-0941-7

Vol. 56 Santiago Pérez Isasi and Ângela Fernandes (eds)
Looking at Iberia. A Comparative European Perspective.
317 pages. 2013.
ISBN 978-3-0343-0934-9

Vol. 57 Daniel de Zubía Fernández
Señas del esplendor ausente. Itinerarios familiares en *Señas de identidad* y en *O Esplendor de Portugal*
373 pages. 2014.
ISBN 978-3-0343-0963-9

Vol. 58 Helena Usandizaga (ed.)
Palimpsestos de la antigua palabra. Inventario de mitos prehispánicos en la literatura latinoamericana
383 pages. 2013.
ISBN 978-3-0343-0967-7

Vol. 59 *Forthcoming*

Vol. 60 Guillermo Laín Corona
Proyecciones de Gabriel Miró en la narrativa del 27.
250 pages. 2013.
ISBN 978-3-0343-0952-3

Vol. 61 Javier Ordiz (ed.)
Estrategias y figuraciones de lo insólito en la narrativa mexicana (siglos XIX–XXI)
237 pages. 2014.
ISBN 978-3-0343-1729-0

Vol. 62 Anna Vives
Identidad en tiempos de vanguardia: narcisismo, genio y violencia en la obra de Salvador Dalí y Federico García Lorca.
323 pages. 2015.
ISBN 978-3-0343-1792-4

Vol. 63 C.A. Longhurst
Modernismo, noventayochismo y novela: España y Europa. Ensayo de literatura comparada.
262 pages. 2014.
ISBN 978-3-0343-1810-5

Vol. 64 *Forthcoming*

Vol. 65 Ángela Gracia Menéndez
Gaspar de Jovellanos: crítico, reformador y humanista ilustrado.
202 pages. 2015.
ISBN 978-3-0343-1849-5

Vol. 66 Michael W. Stannard
Galdós and Medicine.
240 pages. 2015.
ISBN 978-3-0343-1825-9

Vol. 67 Helena Usandizaga y Beatriz Ferrús (eds.)
Fragmentos de un nuevo pasado: inventario de mitos prehispánicos en la literatura latinoamericana actual.
467 pages. 2015.
ISBN 978-3-0343-1852-5